Confusional States in Older People

Eleanor Jane Byrne MRCPsych

Senior Lecturer and Honorary Consultant,
Department of Old Age Psychiatry, University
of Manchester, School of Psychiatry and
Behavioural Sciences, Withington Hospital,
Manchester

Edward Arnold
A member of the Hodder Headline Group
LONDON   BOSTON   MELBOURNE   AUCKLAND

© 1994 E. J. Byrne

First published in Great Britain 1994

Distributed in the Americas by Little, Brown and Company
34, Beacon Street, Boston, MA 02108

British Library Cataloguing in Publication Data

Bryne, E. J.
  Confusional States in Older People
  I. Title
  618.97689

  ISBN 0–340–56298–6

Whilst the advice and information in this book is believed to be
true and accurate at the date of going to press, neither the author
nor the publisher can accept any legal responsibility or liability for
any errors or omissions that may be made.

Typeset in 10/11 pt Times by Anneset, Weston-super-Mare, Avon.
Printed in Great Britain for Edward Arnold, a division of
Hodder Headline PLC, 338 Euston Road, London NW1 3BH by
St Edmunsbury Press Ltd., Bury St Edmunds, Suffolk and bound
by Hunter & Foulis Ltd, Edinburgh.

DEDICATION

To my earliest and best teachers;
Patricia Sarsfield Byrne and Kathleen Marianne Pearson

Preface

Confusional states in older people are common, distressing to those who suffer from them and those who care for them, and a major health problem. Despite this they have been, until relatively recently, a 'cinderella' group of conditions – neglected by many. This book is intended as an introduction to the subject and if at times seems thin on data this is, in part a true reflection of our lack of knowledge.

I am constantly learning from my patients, their carers and my colleagues to whom I am immensely grateful.

I have been lucky to 'sit at the feet' of some wise men and women, including my parents, Professor Pat Byrne and Dr Kathleen Pearson, Sir Douglas Black, Professor John Brochlehurst, Dr John Johnson, Professor Leslie Kiloh, Dr John Sydney Smith, Professor Tom Arie, Dr Anthea Lehmann. Many of the ideas in this book are due to their teaching.

E. Jane Byrne
February 1994

ACKNOWLEDGEMENTS

To Tom Arie for encouragement and his eclectic teaching; to my colleagues Alistair Burns, David Jolley and Sean Lennon for enduring the process and to Anne Day without whose hard work this book would never have been completed.

Contents

Chapter 1 _____

Confusion – description or a diagnosis of a common problem?

Everyone knows what 'confusion' means, yet no one does. A room full of health care professionals will produce almost as many definitions as there are people in the room. If words are for the communication of meaning then 'confusion', in the medical context, signally fails. Simpson (1984), in a questionnaire survey, asked 274 doctors and nurses to choose from a list of symptoms and signs of 'confusion' those which they felt were characteristic of the 'state'. He found a great variability in the symptoms and signs that were chosen, from disorientation to anxiety and concluded that the word should not be used unless clearly defined.

Yet the word 'confusion' *is* widely used. Roberts and Caird (1990) probably reflect the majority view in the following:

> *'The term confusion has been used by us to describe the state of patients who showed varying degrees of disorientation for time, place and person, inability to concentrate, short-term memory loss and cognitive decline. It is a useful label because it describes in simple terms, a dominant problem which affects both patients and carers. Its use in initial assessment deliberately precludes attachment of labels such as dementia, which suggests irreversibility, and delirium which suggest reversibility, too early in the course of a patient's illness, at a time when more detailed formulation may well be difficult and prejudicial. The syndrome of confusion cannot always be equated with a diffuse organic brain syndrome and careful clinical evaluation is required.'*

I will attempt to show in this book that the distinction between the well validated syndromes, dementia and delirium, is not only possible but important and that perhaps we as doctors are more afraid of 'labels' than our patients or their carers.

The meaning of 'confusion'

The word confusion has been used as a diagnosis, 'she suffers from confusion': as a syndrome (see above); and as a descriptive term ('she has dementia characterized by severe confusion'). As a diagnosis it is incomplete, and surely it is difficult consistently to recognize a syndrome if no-one can agree as to its features. Throughout this book I will take the definition of Lishman (1987): 'confusion is a descriptive term meaning thinking with less than accustomed clarity'. In this sense it is a feature of many common syndromes whose cause may be either organic or functional.

Confusional states

Like the word 'confusion, the term 'confusional states' is purely descriptive and describes those states, some of which are syndromes and some of which are diseases, in which 'thinking with less than accustomed clarity' – confusion – is a feature. To add to the terminological disagreements, many of these states have a number of different synonyms, as shown in Table 1.1.

In clinical practice some of the terminological disagreement becomes almost redundant. We are faced with confusional states in a number of different contexts – the surgery, the outpatient department, on hospital wards – in these contexts what often determines our management is not what we call a state, but the time course that is has run. That at least is the approach that I have

Table 1.1 Synonyms used for some of the confusional states

Delirium	Acute confusional state
	Acute organic brain syndrome
	Acute brain failure
	Toxic confusion
	Pharmacotoxic psychosis
	Acute organic psychosis
	Acute organic reaction
	Metabolic encephalopathy
	Cerebral insufficiency syndrome
	Exogenous psychosis
	Pseudosenility
	Reversible cognitive dysfunction confusion
	Acute agitated delirium
	Dysergastic reaction
Dementia	Chronic confusional state
	Chronic organic brain syndrome
	Chronic brain failure
	Chronic organic reaction
Sub-acute confusional state	
	Sub-acute amnesic syndrome
	Acute confusional state
Depression	Major depression
	Affective disorder
	Uni-polar depression
Schizophrenia	Late paraphrenia
	Paranoid state of late onset
	Paraphrenia

taken in this book. This does not mean that I consider that a full description of the state is not important, whatever the context. Indeed, I believe that management decisions flow logically from an initial assessment, as long as that assessment is careful and does not neglect fundamental clinical skills. What is of supreme importance, in my view, is that we make the attempt to distinguish between the different types of confusional state, from the moment that we are first confronted by the problem and are not satisfied with the catch-all phrase 'confusion' as the end result of our initial assessment. I would go so far as to say that those who conclude their initial assessment with nothing more in the way of a diagnosis than the word 'confusion' (unqualified), are thinking with less than accustomed clarity. That is not to say that the distinction between these states is always easy, but a careful clinical approach, utilizing a clinical method which is universal, will increase the likelihood of doing so and, at the very least, will provide a basis for further elucidation of the problem. That it is possible to distinguish between the 'confusional' states has been shown in a number of studies. For example, Seltzer and Sherwin (1978) re-examined 80 patients in a veterans hospital in the United states who had received a non-specific diagnosis such as organic brain syndrome or organic psychosis and found that precise diagnosis, such as multi-infarct dementia, or herpes simplex encephalitis could be made in all but three of these. They also found that 12 of the 80 cases (15%) had functional psychiatric disorders which of course are potentially treatable.

Rabins and Folstein 1982 validated the distinction between delirium and dementia, on phenomenological grounds and found that this was supported by differences in physiological factors such as cardiovascular factors (demented patients had higher blood pressure (BP) both systolic and diastolic) and EEG findings (delirious patients had more diffusely slow records than demented patients). Follow-up of their subjects showed delirium to have a higher mortality rate than dementia at one year follow-up, with both 'confusional states' having higher mortality rates than non-cognitively impaired individuals from the same population.

This book will concentrate on the confusional states which are due to physical disease – *delirium* (acute confusional state) and *dementia* (chronic confusional state). Other confusional states will be considered as differential diagnoses.

Epidemiology of confusional states in elderly people

Confusional states in elderly people are common, in most settings, home, general practice surgery and hospital. It is not surprising that they have been described as 'the silent epidemic', and one of the 'greats' of geriatric medicine. In describing the epidemiology of these states I have tried to indicate how commonly each is found in different settings. All literature reported uses standardized diagnostic assessments and operational definitions. The studies, when compared, are those which have used similar methods. No epidemiological study in this area is perfect but hopefully this represents a selection of the most accurate to date.

Delirium

There is very little data on the prevalence of delirium in the community. One large epidemiological study of mental disorders in Boston, USA (Folstein et al., 1991) found six cases of delirium in the total population who were intensively screened (810). All these individuals were aged 56 years or more. The prevalence of delirium in this study for those aged 55 years or more was 1.08%. Delirium in these six community cases was associated with multiple medications (6/6), visual impairment (4/6), diabetes (4/6), brain disease (4/6) incontinence (3/6) and diuretic use (3/6).

Nursing home residents have been evaluated, but the results are often reported as 'organic' states, undifferentiated into delirium, dementia or other organic syndromes. In two studies from the United States (Rovner et al., 1986; Bienenfield and Wheeler, 1989), delirium was found in six per cent of residents (in one of these studies the diagnostic criteria were not given). Most of the information on the prevalence of delirium comes from hospital studies. Several important observations arise from such surveys; first, there is a serious under-diagnosis of delirium in elderly people in hospital; second, delirious patients have a higher mortality rate than non-delirious patients, thirdly delirium is associated with serious physical illness and certain conditions (or operative procedures) have a high risk of delirium.

1. *Under-diagnosis of delirium* Most authors have concluded that this is due to two main factors; the failure to recognize delirium in hypoalert patients and the over-reliance on cross-sectional assessments of cognitive status (if such assessment is made at all).
2. *High Mortality rates for delirium* This is almost certainly due to the seriousness of the associated physical illness(es). Death follows delirium, within one month in between 15 per cent and 40 per cent of cases. This is about twice as high as the death rate in similar hospital populations of non-delirious patients. The morbidity of delirious patients is also higher than that of non-delirious patients; they tend to have longer lengths of hospital admissions and a higher mortality rate at three and six months.

Prevalence of delirium in hospital populations

The prevalence of delirium in various hospital populations (of those aged 65 years or more) is shown in Table 1.2. These prevalence rates are the ranges from those published in the literature in studies using operational diagnostic criteria. (The exception is the multi-centre study of Hodkinson, 1973 who used mental test score and decline cognition within two weeks or assessment as criteria for 'confusion'). Lipowski (1992) has concluded that 'at least one in four elderly people admitted to a general hospital will display delirium at some point during their stay'.

Table 1.2 Prevalence of delirium (in people aged 55 years or more) in hospital populations.

	Type of population	Prevalence (%)
Medicine	General medicine	15.1–16.3
	*Geriatric Medicine	24
	Old age psychiatry	13
Surgery	Heart	32
	Hip	28–61
	Orthopaedic	26

*Non-operational diagnostic criteria.
Sources:
General Medicine: Erkinjuntti et al. (1986); Francis et al. (1990); Johnson et al. (1990); Rockwood (1989)
Geriatric Medicine: Hodkinson (1973)
Old-age psychiatry: Kaponen (1989)
Heart: Smith and Dimsdale (1989)
Hip: Berggren et al. (1987); Gustafson et al. (1988)
Orthopaedic: Rogers et al. (1989)

Dementia

Prevalence of dementia

Much more information is available about the prevalence of dementia in old people living at home. Figure 1.1 shows the age specific prevalence rates of old people living at home in Europe. These prevalence rates are the averages from the Eurodem project (Hofman et al., 1991). It can be seen that dementia before the age of 65 years is very rare, but thereafter the prevalence rate doubles every five years.

From the same data set the prevalences of Alzheimer type dementia and vascular dementia, in old people living at home in Europe are shown in Figures 1.2–1.4. Although the prevalence rates for Alzheimer's disease

Fig. 1.1   Age specific prevalence of dementia (all types) in Europe

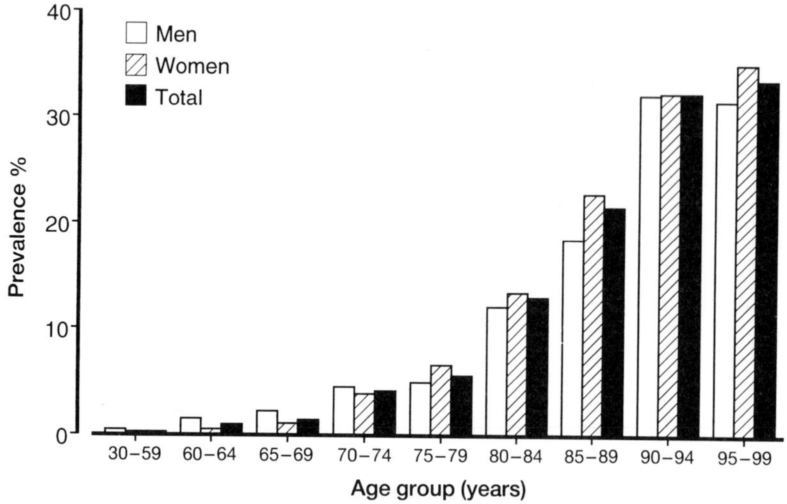

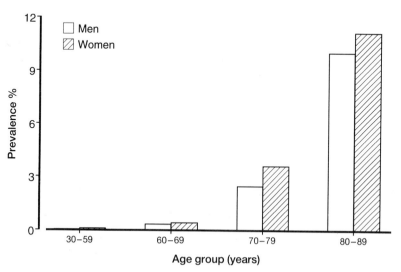

Source: Hofman et al. (1991).

Source: Rocca et al. (1991a).

Fig. 1.2   Age specific prevalence of Alzheimer's disease in Europe.

Fig. 1.3   Age specific prevalence of vascular dementia in men in Europe

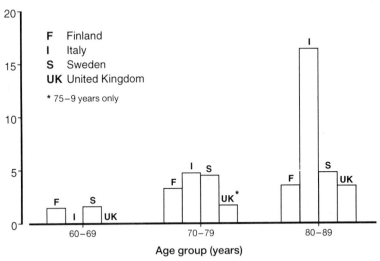

Source: Rocca et al. (1991b).

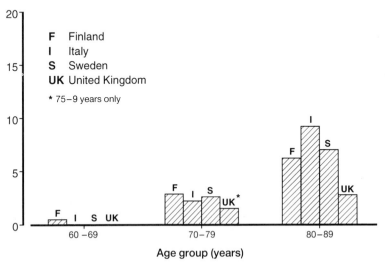

Source: Rocca et al. (1991b).

Fig. 1.4   Age specific prevalence of vascular dementia in women in Europe

Fig. 1.5   Age specific incidence of dementia in Nottingham

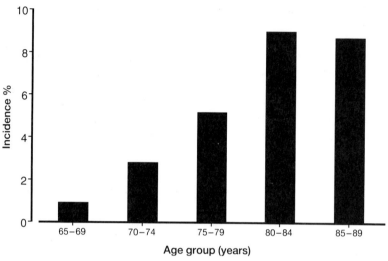

Source: Morgan et al. (1992).

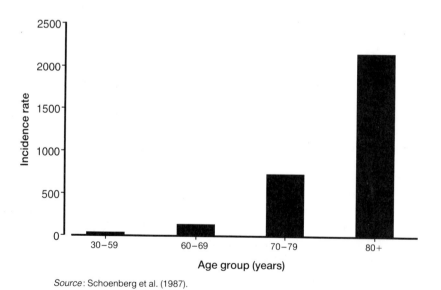

Source: Schoenberg et al. (1987).

Fig. 1.6   Age specific incidence (per 100,000) in Rochester, Minnesota, USA

(AD) are quite uniform across Europe, those for vascular dementia especially among men, show wide differences between countries. This may reflect true geographical differences in the prevalence of vascular dementia, or may be due to inclusion of mixed dementia (AD and vascular dementia in the same patient), amongst those designated as 'cases'.

The diagnosis of vascular dementia is notoriously inaccurate, but the epidemiology of stroke disease also shows great variation by prevalence between countries across the world, therefore true geographical differences in the prevalence of vascular dementia cannot be ruled out.

In the United States age specific prevalence of dementia (undifferentiated) is 65–74 years 1.1 per cent, 75–84 years 4.3 per cent and 85 years or more 16.8 per cent (Weissman et al., 1985). The age-specific incidence per 100,000 of the population in the USA is shown in Fig 1.6.

Prevalence of dementia in other settings

The prevalence of Dementia is, perhaps not surprisingly, higher in both hospital and residential home populations of old people. In hospital, about 40 per cent of admissions to geriatric medical wards are found to have dementia on admission, of these about 25 per cent will also have delirium (Hodkinson et al., 1973). On general medical wards, one large study found the prevalence of dementia to range from 0.8 per cent of those aged 55–64 years to 31.2 per cent of those aged more than 85 years. The prevalence for the total population aged 55 years or more was 9.1 per cent. (Erkinjuntti et al., 1986).

Elderly people are the greater consumers of health care (OECD, 1988) than the non-elderly population therefore it is to be expected that significant proportions of old people will present to all types of services. There is little information on the prevalence of confusional state in other hospital departments such as Accident and Emergency.

In residential care for the elderly the range of the prevalence figures for dementia (as might be expected) is very wide from 25–75 per cent in nursing homes (Henderson 1992) to 67 per cent of Part III residents (Mann et al., 1984). On the whole, rest home residents are less impaired than nursing home residents but dementia is still common in rest homes.

In general practice elderly patients have been identified from age - sex registers and screened by researchers. In one such study which included 6 general practices 444 out of 2616 (91 per cent of all those in the register) patients screened were examined in detail (O'Connor et al 1988) 96 (22 per cent) were found to have 'mild' dementia 85 (19 per cent) had 'moderate' dementia, 27 (6 per cent) had 'severe' dementia, and 236 (53 per cent) were not demented.

Incidence of dementia

The age specific incidence of dementia (from Nottingham) is shown in Fig. 1.5. This study suggests, that for an average Health District (population 250,000 with 15 per cent age over 65 years) there will be around 700 new cases of dementia each year. Incidence studies also provide information about potential risk factors for the development of dementia. In the Nottingham, UK study, only analgesics used as a hypnotic was confirmed as a risk factor for dementia of those factors examined (handedness, heart disease, giddiness, falls, headaches, smoking, insomnia, hypnotic use other sleep medicines).

Van Duijun et al 1991, have reviewed 11 case-control studies from around the world which assess risk factors for Alzheimer's disease. Family history of dementia, Down's syndrome and Parkinson's disease were all significant risk factors for AD.

Conclusion

Confusional states in old people are common in many different settings. It is possible and desirable to distinguish between the confusional states in old age.

References

Berggren, D., Gustafson, Y., Eriksson, B., Bacht, C., Harrison, L.I., Reiz, S. and Winblad, B. (1987). Postgeriatric confusion after anaesthesia in elderly patients with femoral neck fractures. *Anesthesia and Analgesia*. **66**: 497–504.

Bienefield, D. and Wheeler, B.G. (1989). Psychiatric services to nursing homes: a liaison model. *Hospital and Community Psychiatry*. **40**: 793–794.

Erkinjuntti, T., Wikstraun, J., Polo, J. and Aetio, L. (1986). Dementia among medical in-patients evaluation of 2000 consecutive admissions. *Archives of Internal Medicine*. **146**: 1923–1926.

Francis, J., Martin, D. and Kapoor, W.N. (1991). A prospective study of delirium in hospitalised elderly. *Journal of the American Medicine Association*. **263**: 1097–1101.

Folstein, M.F., Bassett, S.S., Romanoski, A.J., Nestadt, G. (1991). The epidemiology of delirium in the community: the Eastern Baltimore Mental Health Survey. *International Psychogeriatrics*. **3**: 169–176.

Gustafson, Y., Berggren, D., Branstram, B., Bacht, G., Norberg, A., Hanson, L.I., Winblad, B. (1988). Acute confusional states in elderly patients treated for femoral neck fracture. *Journal of the American Geriatrics Society*. **36**: 525–530.

Henderson, A.S. (1992). The epidemiology of mental illness. In *Oxford Text Book of Geriatric Medicine*. Evans, J.G. and Williams, T.F. (eds). Oxford: Oxford University Press, pp. 617–620.

Hofman, A, Rocca, W.A., Brayne, C. et al. (1991). The prevalence of dementia in Europe: A collaborative study of 1980–1990 findings. *International Journal of*

Epidemiology. **20**: 736–748.

Hodkinson, H.M. (1973). Mental impairment in the elderly. *Journal of the Royal College of Physicians London*. **7**: 305–317.

Johnson, J., Gottlieb, G.L., Sullivane, Wanich, C., Kinosian, B., Forciea, M. A., Sims, R. and Hogue, C. (1990). Using DSM III criteria to diagnose delirium in elderly medical in-patients. *Journal of Gerontology and Medical Sciences*. **45**, M113–116.

Kaponen, H., Stenback, H., Mattila, F., Solrinen, H., Reinlkainen, K. and Riekkinen, P.J. (1989). Delirium among elderly patients admitted to the psychiatric hospital clinical course during the acute stage and one-year follow-ups. *Acta Psychiatrica Scandinavia*. **79**, 579–585.

Levkoff, S., Cleary, P., Liptzin, B. and Evans, D.A. (1991). Epidemiology of delirium: an overview of research issues and findings. *International Psychogeriatrics*. **3**: 179–167.

Lipowski, Z.J. (1992). Delirium and impaired consciousness In *Oxford Text Book of Geriatric Medicine*. Evans, J.E. and Williams, T.F. (eds). Oxford: Oxford University Press, pp. 490–496.

Lishman, W.A. (1987). *Organic Psychiatry*. Oxford: Blackwell.

Mann, A.H., Graham, N. and Ashby, D. (1984). Psychiatric illness in residential homes for the elderly: a survey in one London Borough. *Age and Ageing*. **13**, 257–265.

Morgan, K., Lilley, J., Arie, T., Byrne, E.J., Jonwa, R. and Waite, J. (1992). Incidence of Dementia: preliminary findings from the Nottingham longitudinal study of activity and ageing. *Neuroepidemiology*. **11**: 80–83.

O'Connor, D.W., Pollitt, P.A., Hyde, J.B., Brook, C.P.B., Reiss, B.B. and Roth, M. (1988). Do general practitioners miss dementia in elderly patients. *British Medical Journal*. **297**: 1107–1110.

Rabins, P. and Folstein, M.F., (1982). Delirium and dementias: diagnostic criteria and fatality rates. *British Journal of Psychiatry*. **140**: 149–153.

Roberts, M.A. and Caird, F.I. (1990). The contribution of computerised tomography to the differential diagnosis of confusion in elderly people. *Age and Ageing*. **19**: 50–56.

Rocca, W.A., Hofman, A., Brayne, C. et al. (1991a). Frequency and distribution of Alzheimer's disease in Europe: a collaborative study of 1980–1990 prevalence findings. *Annals of Neurology*. **30**: 381–390.

Rocca, W.A., Hofman, A. and Brayne, C. et al. (1991b). The prevalence of vascular dementia in Europe: facts and fragments from 1980–1990 studies. *Annal of Neurology*. **30**: 817–824.

Rockwood, K. (1989). Acute confusion in elderly medical in-patients. *Journal of the American Geriatrics Society*. **37**: 150–154.

Rogers, M.P., Llong, M.H., Daltray, L.H., Eaton, H., Petect. J., Wright, E. and Albert, M. (1989). Delirium after elective orthopaedic surgery: risk factors and natural history. *International Journal of Psychiatry in Medicine*. **19**: 109–121.

Rovner, B.W., Kafonek, S., Filipp, L., Lucas, M.J., Folstein, M.F. (1986). Prevalence of mental illness in a community nursing home. *American Journal of Psychiatry*. **143**: 1446–1449.

Seltzer, B. and Sherwin, I. (1978). 'Organic brian syndromes': an empirical study and criteria review. *American Journal of Psychiatry*. **135**: 13–21.

Schoenberg, B.S., Kokmen, E. and Okazaki, H. (1987). Alzheimer's disease and other dementing illnesses in a defined United States population: incidence rates and clinical features. *Annals of Neurology*. **22**: 724–729.

Simpson, C.T. (1984). Doctors and nurses use of the word confused. *British Journal of Psychiatry*. **145**: 441–443.

Smith, L.W. and Dimsdale, J.E. (1989). Postcardiotomy delirium. Conclusions after 25 years? *American Journal of Psychiatry*. **146**: 452–458.

Van Duijn, C.M., Stijnen, T. and Hofman, A. (1991). Risk factors for Alzheimer's disease: overview of the EURODEM collaborative re-analysis of case-control studies. *International Journal of Epidemiology*. **20** (Suppl. 2): 54–573.

Weissman, M.M., Myers, J.K., Tischler, G.L., Holtzer, C.E-III, Leaf, P. J., Orvaschel, H. and Brody, J.A. (1985). Psychiatric disorder (DSM-III) and cognitive impairment among the elderly in a US urban community. *Acta Psychiatrica Scandinavica*. **71**: 366–379.

Chapter 2 _____

Delirium (Acute confusional state)

Definition

Delirium may be defined as a 'transient organic mental syndrome of acute onset and featuring concurrent disturbance of consciousness, a global cognitive and attentional disorder. Reduced or increased psychomotor activity, and a disrupted sleep-wake cycle' (Lipowski, 1990). This definition is in line with the major classification systems – DSM-III-R (APA 1987) and ICD 10 (WHO 1992) (see Appendix 2.1) but is concise, a useful 'beside' definition.

Clinical features

Acute onset

There is little data on the time course of delirium in elderly patients, possibly because it is often missed (see Chapter 6). Most patients have a *prodromal stage* lasting from a few hours to a day or so, Morse and Litin (1969) report a prodromal phase in 81% of their patients. Prodromal features are listed in Table 2.1 and consist of a change in the patient's habitual behaviour and cognitive functioning. Relatives or friends may say that the patient became suddenly 'confused' or that they did not seem like their usual self.

Table 2.1 Features of the prodrome of delirium

Sleep disturbance – vivid dreams and/or insomnia
Restlessness and irritability
Difficulty in concentrating and thinking clearly
Increased awareness of sights and sounds
Tiredness or fatiguability
General malaise
Anxiety
Occasionally perceptual abnormalities (illusions or hallucinations)

Source: Lipowski 1990.

It is worth asking such informants for the features listed in Table 2.1. Frequently these are especially noticeable at night time. There is not only a change from the patient's pre-morbid state but change is one of the cardinal features in delirium – the symptoms vary over time and there may be periods of relative lucidity. This is why *history and observation* over time, are of great importance diagnostically. Some patients never progress beyond the prodromal stage, in others the following symptoms, summarized in Table 2.2 become more obvious or more severe.

Table 2.2 Clinical features of delirium (acute confusional state)

Acute onset – hours or few days
Change in symptoms over time – often worse at night
Disturbance in consciousness
Global impairment in cognition
   Memory – registration, recent, remote, sequencing
   Orientation
   Thinking – often dream-like
   Perception – misidentification, hallucinations
Disordered attention
Altered sleep-wake cycle
Altered mood – often anxious or fearful
Altered activity level – hyperactive or hypo-active

Source: Macdonald et al. (1989).

Disturbance of consciousness

It has been traditional in many descriptions of delirium to include the phrase 'clouding of consciousness', yet few are able to describe it, and even fewer to define it. That useful medical instrument the 'retrospectoscope' seems to be the best means of identifying it! Yet in most patients at some point in their delirium abnormalities in consciousness can be observed. The patient may be awake but seems distractible and to have difficulty in interpreting environmental stimuli. They seem to drift in and out of awareness of their surroundings and this communication is fragmentary and changeable. At times there is an appropriate response to a question, at others they seem not to have heard what was said or are distracted by even the slightest noise such as the ticking of a clock. It is as if the normal filtering mechanism we all employ in everyday life to avoid being bombarded by extraneous stimuli has broken down. A good example of the filter at work is a tannoy system in a hospital. Doctors are able to ignore the constant stream of announcements unless it has immediate personal significance such as their names being called. Similarly, on a holiday beach we are able to ignore the radios, children playing, until someone inadvertently steps on our toes. We respond to the tannoy system or the tread on our toes according to our past experience and our personality, but in both cases there is a considered response – we are immediately alert – we have correctly identified an incoming stimulus and respond appropriately. The delirious patient is, however, unable either to identify the incoming stimulus or to use past experience or to focus attention in order to respond. Neither can they overcome these difficulties by voluntary effort.

Global impairment of cognitive function

Cognition is generally held to refer to all processes that are employed in information processing – that is, perceiving, remembering, thinking and imagining (Lipowski, 1990)

Perceptual abnormalities

These range from misidentification of people or objects, to a delirious patient – the coat hanging behind the door appears as if it is a man standing in a threatening posture – to full-blown hallucinations in any modality, but most commonly visual or auditory. Visual hallucinations are traditionally held to occur in organic rather than functional states. They do occur in the latter and so are unreliable on their own as a diagnostic feature. It is their occurrence with the other features of delirium which gives significance. They are very common in delirium being found in between 15% and 70% of cases. The patient may be seen trying to brush the 'ants' off their bed and hallucinations are sometime inferred by such observations rather than the patient reporting their presence.

Memory

Both recent and remote memory are impaired. The patient is unable to remember important events in their life, nor what they were doing the previous day, or even 2 minutes ago.
Even if there is recall of life events (in a period or relative lucidity) they will usually be recalled in the wrong order – a time sequencing problem.

Orientation

The usual sequence in formal testing of orientation is time, place and person. This is the order in which they are lost in both delirium and dementia. A variety of disorientation for place is described in some detail by Max Levin (1968), a physician who suffered from delirium during the course of a serious illness.

> *'My wife . . . told me that I was in the Presbyterian Hospital. Thenceforth I always knew where I was but had a remarkable misconception of the location of the hospital in relation to my home . . . I knew that I was in the hospital, but I believed the hospital had a small branch . . . less than a mile from my home; I thought I was in this branch. I visualised the path from home to this branch'.*

This phenomena is called geographical disorientation.

Thinking

There is disturbance of normal thought processes, which are usually continuous, organized, conceptual and rich in content. In delirium the patient's thinking is chaotic and often has a dream-like quality. The patient's thoughts may be impoverished, or dominated by abnormal perceptual experiences, hallucinations or misidentifications, and by delusional ideas which are often paranoid. The misidentification of the coat on the back of the door as a threatening man may become incorporated into a false belief that anyone who approaches is part of a sinister conspiracy.

Disorder of attention

It is not uncommon for the clinician interviewing a patient with delirium to have the feeling that the patient is drifting in and out of awareness. This may partly be due to disturbance of consciousness, but also to impaired attention. At times the patient may respond promptly and quickly to a question, at others the response is delayed, if it occurs at all the questions frequently have to be repeated several times. The patient is also typically easily distracted by competing stimuli, such as the noise of a clock ticking or someone walking by. The distractibility is due to an inability to focus attention and to ignore 'irrelevant' stimuli (deficient selective attention). Distractibility may also arise from internal events such as hallucinations.

In addition to the difficulty in selective attention, in delirium attention as a more generalised cognitive function, that of the ability to be in a state of readiness to respond to stimuli, is also impaired.

Altered sleep-wake cycle

Day time drowsiness and nocturnal wakefulness is not an uncommon alteration in the sleep-wake cycle in delirium. Indeed, so common is the phenomenon of nocturnal worsening of delirium that some advocate this feature as a cardinal diagnostic sign. This observation has also led to some of the common suggestions for the management of the delirious patient at night time; leaving lights on, to reduce the misidentifications and misinterpretations of stimuli, or playing a radio.

Although there is no objective evidence that these strategies are either appropriate or successful. It is important to note that alterations in the sleep-wake cycle are as variable as the course of the delirium itself; at times they may be prominent at others this may not be a noticeable feature.

Altered mood

May be a feature of the prodrome or the syndrome proper. Fear, anxiety and depression are the commonest alterations of mood. The fearfulness may be unfocused on real or psychotic events. For example, the illusion of a person standing behind a door, due to misinterpretation of a coat which is hanging there, may lead to the fear that someone is going to harm them. Clinical manifestations of anxiety (somatic anxiety) may accompany the fear (psychic anxiety), the person may look anxious, be restless or fidgety, have a rapid pulse and sweaty palms.

Depression may be quite intense, at times leading to suicidal attempts. Unlike idiopathic depressive illness, however, the depressed mood in delirium is not sustained over time, that is, it is not evident throughout the delirium, and again unlike depressive illness may be most obvious at night. Most often depressed mood is variable, at times the patient is weepy and expressing gloomy thoughts, at others no abnormality of mood is shown.

Less commonly, the mood change may resemble mania, with excessive cheerfulness, mixed with irritability and suspiciousness.

Altered activity level

The level of activity in patients with delirium may be increased or decreased and is usually variable although some patients may be consistently over-active and others under-active. The level of activity often mirrors the other features of delirium, for example when the patient is floridly deluded and experiencing hallucinations, experiences usually associated with a fearful affect, they are usually behaviourally over-active. One possible reason why the diagnosis of delirium is so often missed is the lowered activity levels of some delirious patients. They lie quietly out of touch with their surroundings and so do not draw attention to themselves. This is particularly true in busy hospital wards.

Pathophysiology of delirium

The exact nature of the pathophysiology of delirium is unknown. Both cortical and brain-stem functions are impaired in delirium, the cortex mediating cognitive function and the brain-stem wakefulness. It is likely that these changes are the result of neurotransmitter abnormalities, especially acetyl choline. The neurotransmitter abnormalities themselves may be produced by a variety of mechanisms which can be subsumed under two main headings; *blood brain barrier deficits*, which is an abnormality that could lead to the leakage of drugs or other toxins into the brain tissue; *altered metabolism*, which could be generalized as in anoxia or specific as in thalamic lesions.

Sub-types of delirium

There is some clinical and electro-encephalographic evidence for the subdivision of delirium into two types, acute delirium (acute confusional state) and sub-acute delirium (sub-acute confusional state) (Engel and Romano, 1959; Mori and Yamadori, 1987). The similarities and differences are show in Table 2.3. However, in a large number of cases patients have features of both types probably reflecting the characteristic fluctuation of delirium. Liptzin and Levkoff (1992) have shown that sub-types can be identified in elderly (age 65 years or more) hospital patients but found that the mixed type was commonest in their sample. In this study the hyperactive type had the best outcome and they suggest that these patients may command more medical and nursing attention. These sub-types require further validation.

Table 2.3 Similarities and differences between acute and sub-acute confusional states

Acute confusional state (hyperactive)	Sub-acute confusional state (hypoactive)
Similarities Clouding of consciousness Global impairment of cognition Fluctuation of symptoms	
Differences	
Acute onset (hours or day)	Less acute onset (days or weeks)
Florid symptoms	Few or no florid symptoms
Usually aroused	Usually not aroused
Brief course (a week or so)	More protracted course (weeks)

Risk factors for delirium

Age, pre-existing brain damage and pre-existing dementia (whatever the aetiology) are factors which predispose to delirium (Lipowski, 1990). Others, such as sensory impairment, may act as maintaining or enhancing factors (see Beresin, 1988). Levkoff et al., 1988 have identified four additional risk factors: urinary tract infection, low serum albumin, raised white cell count, protein and urea. (The latter three are included in the absence of preceding factors.) A number of studies have established risk factors for delirium following surgery (see Whitaker, 1989) these include age, previous alcohol or drug abuse, and prolonged operations.

APPENDIX 1

DSM III-R criteria for delirium.
A. Reduced ability to maintain attention at external stimuli (e.g. questions must be repeated because attention wanders) and to appropriately shift

attention to a new external stimuli (e.g. perseverates answer to a previous question).

B. Disorganized thinking, as indicated by rambling, irrelevant, or incoherent speech.

C. At least two of the following:

reduced level of consciousness, e.g. difficulty keeping awake during examination;
perceptual disturbances: misinterpretations, illusions, or hallucinations;
disturbance of sleep-wake cycle with insomnia or daytime sleepiness;
increased or decreased psychomotor activity;
disorientation to time, place, or person;
memory impairment, e.g. inability to learn new material, such as the names of several unrelated objects after five minutes, or remember past events, such as history of current episode of illness.

D. Clinical features develop over a short period of time (usually hours to days) and tend to fluctuate over the course of a day.

E   Either (1) or (2):

evidence from the history, physical examination, or laboratory tests of a specific organic factor (or factors) judge to be aetiological related to the disturbance;
in the absence of such evidence, an aetiologic organic factor can be presumed if the disturbance cannot be accounted for by any nonorganic mental disorder, e.g. Manic Episode accounting for agitation and sleep disturbance.

ICD-10 diagnostic criteria for delirium

For a definite diagnosis, symptoms, mild or severe, should be present in each one of the following areas:

1. impairment of consciousness and attention (on a continuum from clouding to coma; reduced ability to direct, focus, sustain, and shift attention);

2. global disturbance of cognition (perceptual distortions, illusions and hallucinations – most often visual' impairment of abstract thinking and comprehension, with or without transient delusions, but typically with some degree of incoherence; impairment of immediate recall and of recent memory but with relatively intact remote memory; disorientation for time as well as, in more severe cases, for place and person);

3. psychomotor disturbances (hypo- or hyperactivity and unpredictable shifts from one to the other; increased reaction time; increased or decreased flow of speech; enhanced startle reaction);

4. disturbance of the sleep–wake cycle (insomnia or, in severe cases, total sleep loss or reversal of the sleep–wake cycle; daytime drowsiness; nocturnal worsening of symptoms; disturbing dreams or nightmares, which may continue as hallucinations after awakening);

5. emotional disturbances, e.g. depression, anxiety or fear, irritability, euphoria, apathy, or wondering perplexity.

References

American Psychiatric Association (1987). *Diagnostic and Statistical Manual of Mental Disorders*, 3rd edn. Washington DC. American Psychiatric Association.

Beresin, E. V. (1988). Delirium in the elderly. *Journal of Geriatric Psychiatry and Neurology*. **1**: 127–143.

Engel, G. L. and Romano, J. (1959). Delirium: a syndrome of cerebral insufficiency. *Journal of Chronic Diseases*. **9**: 260–277.

Levin, M. (1968) Delirium: an experience and some reflections. *American Journal of Psychiatry*. **124**: 1120.

Levkoff, S. E., Safron, C., Cleary, P. D., Gallop, J. and Phillips, R. S. (1988). Identification of factors associated with the diagnosis of delirium in elderly hospitalised patients. *Journal of the American Geriatric Society*. **36**: 1099–1104.

Lipowski Z. J. (1990). *Delirium: Acute Confusional States*. New York: Oxford University Press.

Liptzin, B and Levkoff, S. E. (1992). An empirical study of delirium sub-types. *British Journal of Psychiatry*. **161**: 843–845.

Macdonald, A. J. D., Simpson, A. and Jenkins, D. (1989). Delirium in the elderly: a review and a suggestion for a research programme. *International Journal of Geriatric Psychiatry*. **4**: 311–319.

Mori, E. and Yamadoria, A. (1987). Acute confusional state and acute agitated delirium. Occurrence after infarction of the right middle cerebral artery. *Archives of Neurology*. **44**: 1139–1143.

Morse, R. M. and Litin, E. M. (1969) Post-operative delirium: a study of aetiologic factors. *American Journal of Psychiatry*. **126**: 388–395.

Whitaker, J. J. (1989). Postoperative confusion in the elderly. *International Journal of Geriatric Psychiatry*. **4**: 321–326.

World Health Organisation, (1992). *Manual of the International Statistical Classification of Diseases, Injuries and Cause of Death*. 10th edn. Geneva: World Health Organisation

Chapter 3 _____

Dementia

Definitions

Dementia has been described as, 'An acquired, global impairment of intellect, memory and personality' Lishman (1987). Such a definition, however, does not convey the essence of the problem that is, dementia. It is deficient in the same way that the telephone exchange analogy inadequately describes the brain, in that it fails to convey the complex and changing ways that damage to a person's brain affects the individual and those around them. There are many definitions of the dementia syndrome. These can be classified into: descriptive (see Appendix 3.1) and operational (where certain conditions have to be fulfilled in order to be given the syndrome diagnosis). Two of the most widely used operational diagnostic criteria are DSM-III R and (see Appendix 3.1) ICD 10.

Most operational definitions place great emphasis on the cognitive features of the dementia syndrome. While this may be of prime diagnostic importance, it is often the non-cognitive features such as depression or behavioural abnormalities that are most troublesome to the sufferer and to those who care for them.

Clinical features

The clinical features of the dementia syndrome are summarized in Table 3.1. Not all the causes of the dementia syndrome will show all of these features.

Cognitive abnormalities

Memory impairment

Many of us have had the experience of going into a room and forgetting what we had gone there for. We remember eventually, although we sometimes have to jog our memory by retracing our footsteps and starting again. Early difficulties with memory in dementia can resemble this forgetfulness, but the ability to respond to 'cues' or jogging of the memory is lost.

Sufferers become more and more forgetful, especially of events that have

Table 3.1 Clinical features of dementia.

Cognitive abnormalities
Memory impairment

Demonstrable evidence of impairment of both short and long term memory

Impairment in abstract thinking
Impaired judgement
Impaired higher cortical
Function (aphasia, apraxia, agnosia, constructional ability)
Personality change

(The cognitive impairments interfere with work or usual social activities, or relationships with others and do not occur exclusively in the course of delirium)

Non-cognitive abnormalities
Disorders of perception (hallucinations, misidentifications)
Disorders of mood
Delusions

Disorders of behaviour
Wandering
Aggression
Inappropriate behaviour
Restlessness

---

happened recently. They may remember clearly details of their life history, landmarks like children's birthdays, when they married and names of long-standing friends, while they forget appointments and cannot remember the lady who came to tea last week. Often they develop ways to cover up the problem. Some patients write appointments down in a notebook, but then forget to look at the entries. When confronted by questions that they cannot answer, they may make gestures to indicate that the answer is on the tip of their tongue; become angry, 'don't bother me with silly questions', or scornful, 'everyone knows what happened'. Gradually they lose their grasp on current events and may appear to dwell in the past. These difficulties are often highlighted by a change in surroundings.

Long-term memory is also impaired (although often this occurs after the recent memory problem), sufferers begin to forget the order in which events occurred in their lives and eventually they forget the events themselves. For example they may forget they are married and refer to their bemused spouse as 'my friend' or 'the lodger'.

Impairment in abstract thinking

Patients with dementia often have difficulty in defining words and concepts which goes beyond the often associated naming difficulties. They are prone to literal interpretation of abstract concepts, so called concrete thinking. In everyday life these deficits may partly explain actions such as putting salt in the cup of tea instead of sugar. This action may be a sequencing error or a problem of recognition, but may also be due to an inability to recognize that all white granular substances are not sugar.

Impaired higher cortical functions

Dysphasia
One problem commonly faced by carers is the difficulty of communication with people who have dementia. Being able to communicate effectively depends on having something to say and then being able to put those thoughts into words. In dementia not only do people have less to say, in that their fund of ideas is diminished, but they also find it difficult to find the right words.

One of the earliest difficulties with speech in dementia is loss of the ability to identify objects by their proper names, although the patient may be aware of their nature or significance. For example, when asked to name a watch the patient may say it is for telling the time. Eventually their speech becomes either less spontaneous and contains fewer words (non-fluent aphasia) or flows freely but contains many words which are used inappropriate so that the listener has great difficulty in understanding what is said (fluent aphasia).

Apraxia
Apraxia is the inability to perform movements when asked by someone else to do so, for example they may be unable to brush their hair, although one can observe them later smoothing it with their hand. A more dramatic example of this symptom is difficulty with dressing or undressing. The patient may put the clothes on upside-down, back-to-front, put their legs into the arms of garments or put clothes on in a bizarre sequence.

Agnosia
The patient may similarly have difficulty in recognizing different parts of their body, and in particular where they lie in relation to each other. Some patients may become muddled as to which is the right side of their body and which is the left. This left-right disorientation may be involved in the dressing difficulty outlined above. Eventually there may be difficulty in recognizing faces of well known friends or family.

Constructional apraxia
Constructional apraxia is the inability to assemble objects in their correct spatial relationship to each other. It is manifest clinically in the inability to perform activities such as laying the table or changing a plug, or to perform simple graphical tasks such as copying a triangle or drawing a house. Examples

of inaccuracies in the clock drawing test in patients with dementia (of varying aetiologies) are shown in Fig. 3.1 and 3.2.

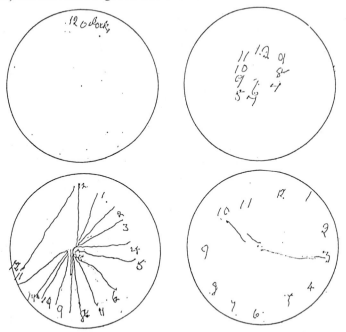

Fig. 3.1   Clock. Drawing Test in Dementia (Varying aetiologies)

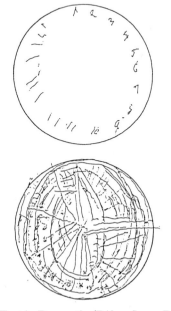

Fig. 3.2   Clock. Drawing Test in Dementia (Difuse Lewy Body Disease)

Personality change

This may be of two main types; an exaggeration of previous character traits, or a complete change from that individual's former habitual 'state of being'. For example the habitually suspicious individual, the kind of person who feels that the world may be against them, begins to believe that it is the case and finds evidence from seemingly trivial occurrences. In some the main personality change is in altered patterns of behaviour, such as the previously respected citizen who begins to use foul language in public.

Judgement

Dementia sufferers are unable to deduce the consequences of their own actions or to make appropriate judgement on how to organize their lives. For example they may wander into a busy dual-carriageway road seemingly unconcerned of the potential risk to life and limb, or be unaware that their lack of self-care has alienated some of those around them. There are of course degrees of impairment of judgement. Clinicians are often asked to help in the decision as to when the dementia sufferer's judgement is sufficiently impaired to warrant overruling what is normally each patient's autonomy or self-determination. This thorny problem will be dealt with later; suffice it to say now that a diagnosis of dementia is not synonymous with a lack of the right to self-determination. Related to judgement is lack of insight into the illness. Some patients are not only unaware of their increasing difficulties but also unconcerned by them. Perhaps equally common, however, are patients who are distressed by them. This awareness may be transitory and lack depth but seems nevertheless to be a painful experience to that person. Anxiety about their own abilities is common, with patients constantly seeking reassurance and panicking if something goes wrong. When faced by a problem they may respond with an explosion of agitation and distress, the 'catastrophic reaction'.

Non-cognitive abnormalities

These common features of the dementia syndrome have, until recently, been neglected by researchers (Burns et al., 1990). Their appearance is, to an extent, dependent on the underlying cause of the dementia syndrome, depression for example is very common in Parkinson's disease and vascular dementia, but most causes of dementia may be associated with non-cognitive abnormalities.

Disorders of perception

Hallucinations in any sensory modality but especially visual and auditory may occur and can be particularly troublesome to the patient; they may also be very difficult to treat. Visual hallucinations may be simple (specks of coloured light, or moving lines) or complex (faces, galloping horses or complete orchestras). Visual hallucinations are more common in patients with impaired vision but are also a feature of some types of dementia, such as diffuse Lewy body disease and Alzheimer's disease (AD) (where they occur in about 10 per cent of patients (Burns et al., 1990). Auditory hallucinations are usually of voices making comments, rarely are they as complex as in schizophrenia.

Illusions, where the patient perceives an object as if it were something else, may also occur in dementia, thus bushes outside the front room window hide predatory strangers. It is not uncommon for illusions and hallucinations to occur in the same patient. The patient's reaction to these experiences is not always one of fear or anguish, one may also observe a partial adaption to the phenomena, as when the sufferer puts down bowls of milk for 'the cat' or lays the table for 'visitors'. The unpleasant nature of the experiences predominates, however, and it is not uncommon for patients to lay traps for the intruders or to keep sticks, scissors or knives around the house for self-defence in the event of attack.

Misidentification where the persons perception of an object is distorted either in quality, intensity or spatial form, is common in dementia, especially in AD (Burns et al.,1990). This distortion of perception is seen in the 'mirror sign', where the patient fails to recognize their own reflection in a mirror, or in the 'picture sign' where the patient may be observed holding conversations with pictures of people cut out of newspapers or magazines. Another misidentification which may occur is the belief that events on television are occurring in three dimensional space.

Disorders of mood

Disorders of mood–depression, anxiety and rarely mania – are probably the commonest non-cognitive disorder in dementia (see Chapter 4). The relationship between mood disorders and dementia is complex; they can be a feature of the illness, a reaction to the illness or may represent the simultaneous occurrence of two common conditions. The importance of recognizing depression in all its guises can not be overemphasized, it is one of the treatable symptoms of dementia and its presence increases the suffering of an already disabled person.

Delusions

In order to experience delusions, one requires relatively intact cognitive functioning. Delusions in dementia are therefore, often seen in the earlier stages of the disease or take the form of fairly simple 'delusion like' ideas, which are often fragmentary or ill-sustained. Common themes of delusions in dementia are of; theft (possibly related to the memory disorder) where the person believes that someone has been stealing articles from their home, which can alienate carers (both formal and informal) who may be accused; of theft; and the delusional belief that others are going to harm them, leading to an unduly suspicious frame of mind. The more common 'delusion-like' ideas consist of forceful transitory beliefs that someone is going to harm them.

Disorders of behaviour

These are among the most worrying and stressful symptoms of dementia, not so much for the sufferer but their carers. Gilleard (1984) in a large survey of problems faced by carers, found that behavioural abnormalities were not only common but very stressful to carers. Table 3.2. lists some of the behavioural problems which may occur in dementia. A fuller discussion of some of these problems is found in Chapter 10.

Table 3.2 Some behavioural problems arising in the or the dementia syndrome

Wandering	Movement without a purpose, or semi-purposeful
Restlessness	Generalised constant purposeless movement
Inappropriate behaviour	May be social, sexual
Aggression	Verbal or physical, generalised or focal
Lack of safety	Poor judgement and memory lead to hazardous situations
Communication problems	Not only when language is affected, perseveration and memory disorders impair communication
Self-neglect	Poor hygiene, omission of medicines, financial problems
Impaired judgement	Leading to reduced capacity for autonomy

It is important to remember that behaviour does not occur in a vacuum. Some behaviours are only problems in certain situations or when observed by certain individuals. For example, wandering out of a home onto a busy road is certainly a problem, whereas wandering in an elderly mentally sick and infirm (EMSI) home is so commonplace as to be the normal. (see Chapter 10).

Differences between dementia and delirium

Some of the major difference between dementia and delirium are shown in Table 3.3. It can be seen that because the modes of onset and the time-scale, in the majority of cases very different from one another, the diagnosis is helped by attention to basic clinical skills; history taking and longitudinal observation. There are of course exceptions to this general rule. Rarely dementia may have a sudden onset, following a massive stroke, for example, or when due to a transmissible dementia. In both of these cases there are additional clinical signs which will aid diagnosis. Vascular dementia may present with nocturnal worsening of cognition as a prominent feature, but a history will reveal an onset spreading over many months or years. It is not uncommon for dementia and delirium to co-exist, again there will be a history of cognitive impairment proceeding the acute state.

Table 3.3 Differences between dementia and delirium

	Dementia	Delirium
Onset	Usually insidious	Sudden
Duration	Years	Days or weeks
Course	Change (usually) over a long time	Change within hours
Consciousness	Normal	Impaired
Sleep-wake cycle	Sleep reversal may occur late in course	Always disturbed
Physical illness (including adverse drug effects)	May be absent	Always present

Source: Adapted from Lipowski, 1992.

Sub-types of the dementia syndrome

As with delirium, there is now good evidence to subdivide the dementia syndrome into two types, cortical and sub-cortical which have clinical relevance (Cummings and Benson, 1984; Tolosa and Alvarez, 1992; Verma et al., 1991). This subdivision is still controversial as some have argued that subcortical dementia is a misnomer as in their view the cognitive deficits are focal (reflecting damage to subcortical/frontal areas) rather than global (Rogers, 1986). The features of sub-cortical dementias are shown in Table 3.4. Other authors would add a 'negative' component to these features, a lack of disorders of higher cortical function apraxia, agnosia or aphasia. The distinctions between cortical and sub-cortical dementia are summarize in Table 3.5.

While the arguments between the 'splitters' and the 'unifiers' continue, those of us who recognise, at the very least, different patterns of cognitive impairment within the confusional state find the concept useful. For example, recognizing sub-cortical dementia immediately defines the list of aetiological possibilities. Causes of the sub-cortical dementia syndrome are listed in Table 3.6.

Table 3.4 Clinical features of sub-cortical dementia.

Forgetfulness
Impaired manipulation of acquired knowledge
Personality changes inertia apathy, perplexity
Psychomotor slowness
Speech disorders
Commonly motor abnormalities

Source: Adapted from Tolosa and Alvarez, 1992.

Table 3.5 Types of dementia-differences between cortical and sub-cortical dementia

Feature	Cortical	Sub-cortical
Memory	Amnesia, inability to respond to cues	Forgetfulness ability to respond to cues
Speech	Normal	Abnormal
Language	Usually present	Often absent
Speed of cognition	Normal or mild slowing	Very slow
Motor abnormalities	Not present or late	Present and early

Source: Adapted from Friedenberg et al., 1989.

Table 3.6 Causes of sub-cortical dementia

Parkinson's disease
Huntingon's chorea
Progressive supranuclear palsy
Lacunar state
Binswanger's disease
Normal pressure hydrocephalus

APPENDIX 3.1

Descriptive definitions of the dementia syndrome

Author(s)	Definition
Wells (1977)	A clinical syndrome of diffuse cognitive impairment, in the absence of clouding of consciousness.
Royal College of Physicians (1981)	The global impairment of higher cortical functions, including memory, the capacity to solve the problems of day-to-day living, the performance of learned perception, motor skills, all aspects of language and communication, and the control of emotional reactions, in the absence of gross clouding of consciousness. The condition is often progressive, though not necessarily irreversible.
McLean (1987)	An acquired decline in a range of cognitive abilities (including memory, learning, orientation, and attention) and intellectual skills (including abstraction, judgement, comprehension, language usage and calculation), accompanied by alterations in personality and behaviour, which impair daily functioning, social skills and emotional control. These impairments appear in a clear conscientiousness and are not due to other psychiatric disorders or focal organic disease. The condition is usually progressive and often irreversible.

DSM-IIIR diagnostic criteria for dementia

A. Demonstrable evidence of impairment in short- and long-term memory. Impairment in short-term memory (inability to learn new information) may be indicated by inability to remember three objects after five minutes. Long-term memory impairment (inability to remember information that was known in the past) may be indicated by inability to remember past personal information (e.g. what happened yesterday, birthplace, occupation) or facts of common knowledge (e.g. past United States Presidents, well-known dates).

B. At least one of the following:
   (1) impairment in abstract thinking, as indicated by inability to find similarities and differences between related words, difficulty in defining words and concepts, and other similar tasks;
   (2) impaired judgement, as indicated by inability to make reasonable plans to deal with interpersonal, family, and job related problems and issues;
   (3) other disturbances of higher cortical function, such as aphasia (disorder of language), apraxia (inability to carry out motor activities despite intact comprehension and motor function), agnosia (failure to recognize or identify objects despite intact sensory function), and 'constructional difficulty' (e.g. inability to copy three-dimensional figures, assemble blocks, or arrange sticks in specific designs);

(4) personality change, i.e., alteration or accentuation of premorbid traits.

C. The disturbance in A and B significantly interferes with work or usual social activities or relationships with others.

D. Not occurring exclusively during the course of delirium.

E. Either (1) or (2)

    (1) there is evidence from the history, physical examination, or laboratory tests of a specific organic factor (or factors) judged to be aetiologically related to the disturbance;

    (2) in the absence of such evidence, an aetiologic organic factor can be presumed if the disturbance cannot be accounted for by any nonorganic mental disorder, e.g. major depression accounting for cognitive impairment.

References

Burns, A., Jacoby, R. and Levy, R. 1990. Psychiatric phenomena in Alzheimer's disease I- IV. *British Journal of Psychiatry*. **157**: 72–94.

Cummings, J.L. and Benson, D.F. (1984). Sub-cortical dementia review of an emerging concept. *Archives of Neurology*. **41**: 874–878.

Friedenberg, D.L., Van Garp, W.G. and Cummings, J.L. (1989). Sub-cortical disorders. In *Demential Disorders Advances and Prospects*. Katona, D.L.E. (ed.). London: Chapman & Hall, pp 104–141.

Gilleard, C.J. (1984). Dementia in the home: Problems faced by care-givers. In *Living with Dementia*. Gilleard, C.J. Beckenham, Groom Helm. pp. 62–75.

Lipowski, Z.J. (1992). Delirium and impaired consciousness. In Oxford Text book of Geriatric Medicine. Evans, T.G. and Williams, T.F. (eds). Oxford: Oxford University Press, pp. 490–496.

Lishman, W.A. (1987). *Organic Psychiatry*. Oxford: Blackwell.

McLean, S. (1987). Assessing dementia I: Difficulties definitions and differential diagnosis. *Australia and New Zealand Journal of Psychiatry*. **21**: 142–174.

Rogers, D. (1986). Bradyphrenia in Parkinsonism: a historical review. *Psychological Medicine*. **16**: 257–265.

Royal College of Physicians. Committee on Geriatrics (1981). Organic mental impairment in the elderly. *Journal of the Royal College of Physicians*. **15**: 142–167.

Tolosa, E.S. and Alvarez, R. (1992). Differential diagnosis of cortical versus subcortical dementia. *Acta Neurologica Scandinavica*. Suppl. 139: 47–53.

Verma, N.P., Yusko, M.J., Byronic-McClung, B.J., Williams, L.A. (1991). Multidisciplinary validation of two dementia categories. In *Alzheimer's Disease: Basil Mechanisms Diagnosis and Therapeutic Strategies*. Iqbal, R., McLachlan, D.R.C., Winblad, B., Isneuski, H.M. (eds). Chichester, Wiley pp. 13–19.

Wells, C.E. (1977). Diagnostic evaluation and treatment In: *Dementia*. 2nd edn. Wells, C.E. (ed.). Philadelphia, Pa: David, pp. 247–275.

Chapter 4 _____

Other confusional states

Effects of ageing

Cognition may be impaired, although this impairment may not fulfil the syndrome diagnosis of dementia or depression, by a number of conditions in old people.|It is of course important to be aware of the physiological changes in cognition that take place in the aging process. A useful and complete description of these can be found in texts like Woods and Britton (1985), suffice it to say that cognition in old people is characterized by slowness and some inflexibility of learning (although this does not mean that learning does not occur) and impaired remembering, but these problems are compatible with independent existence, whereas those in dementia and delirium are not. There is renewed interest in 'age-associated memory impairment' (Crook, 1990) the study of which may help research and treatment of the dementia syndrome.

These aging changes are mediated partly through the central nervous system (CNS) (reduction in the dendritic connections between neurons, Schiebel and Schiebel, 1978) but partly through the increased occurrence in old age of other factors which may impair cognition. Deafness is at peak prevalence in old age and commonly impairs cognition, often quite profoundly but does not in itself cause the dementia syndrome (Gilhome et al., 1980). Conducting a cognitive test with the aid of a hearing amplification device can transform a 'demented' person to a 'normal' old person in five minutes. Severe physical illness or chronic pain may impair cognition; the old person suffering in these ways may be too weak or tired to respond to questions and may mistakenly be regarded as demented.

Hultsch et al., 1993 in a careful study of the interrelationships between physical health; activity; age and cognition in 484 older adults (mean age 69.2 years) living in the community found that physical health affected information processing (fluid intelligence) rather than knowledge crystallized intelligence. They also found that activity levels were associated with cognitive performance (over a wide range of abilities) the more active, the more able, with this effect being greatest in the oldest subjects. Both physical health and activity level moderated the effect of age on cognitive measures. Table 4.1 lists the main differential diagnoses for dementia and delirium. The differential diagnosis listed in Table 4.1 may mimic either delirium or dementia, except dysmnesic syndrome and organic personality change which do not mimic delirium.

Table 4.1 Differential diagnoses of cognitive impairment in old people

Depression
Mania
Schizophrenia
Anxiety state
Personality disorder
Organic hallucinosis
Frontal lobe syndrome
Dysphasia
Dysmnesic syndrome (Korsakoff's syndrome)
Transient global amnesia
Age-associated memory impairment

Pseudodementia

The term pseudodementia has been used to describe cases of functional psychiatric illness which mimics dementia. As Kiloh wrote in his comprehensive 1961 paper, 'the term is purely descriptive and carries no diagnostic weight'. He went on to emphasize the importance of recognizing the true nature of the illness in such patients who might otherwise be danger of therapeutic neglect. Table 4.2 lists the features that may help to distinguish 'pseudodementia' from dementia.

Table 4.2 Features distinguishing between 'pseudodementia' and dementia

Feature	Pseudodementia	Dementia
Onset and duration of symptoms before presentation	Dated with precision and short duration	Imprecise dating and usually long duration
Post psychiatric history	Common	Unusual
Degree of subjective complaint	Severe and detailed	Absent and vague
Behaviour	Appear concerned Behavioural often not congruent with degree of cognitive impairment	Often unconcerned usually congruent impairment
Examination	Many 'don't know' answers Memory loss recent = remote	'Near-miss' answers more typical memory loss recent > remote

Source: Adapted from Wells (1979).

Depression

Depression in old people is a common condition, being found in about 10 per cent of the population over the age of 65 years (Morgan et al., 1987; Blazer et al., 1987). Severe depression, of the type that may mimic dementia and less commonly delirium is found in about 3 per cent of the population aged 65 years or more.

Depressive symptoms (not fulfilling criteria for 'case' depression) are even more common in old people (Blazer et al., 1987) and are frequently seen in association with physical illness (Cohen-Cole and Stoudmire, 1987). In severe depression the patient may be forgetful (due to poor concentration) and mentally sluggish (due to a slowing down of mental and bodily activity). They may not complain of being sad or unhappy. However careful questioning and close observation may reveal depressive thoughts – a feeling of being a burden to everyone; a conviction that they are a bad or wicked person; a feeling that life is not worth living – or a clear fluctuation in the severity of the condition with maximal impairment in the morning and some improvement as the day progresses. In severe depression weight loss may be profound due to inadequate food intake, and the sleep pattern is altered with the patient commonly waking in the early hours of the morning. A history of previous attacks of depression or a family history of depression and a relatively sudden onset of the mental changes may suggest the diagnosis. It can be very difficult, especially in the older patient, to distinguish between depression and dementia. To complicate the matter further, depressive symptoms are not uncommon in people with dementia (Table 4.3). Sometimes the diagnosis only becomes clear when anti-depressant therapy is given.

Table 4.3 Prevalence of depression in some of the major causes of the dementia syndrome

Cause of dementia	Prevalence of depression (%)
Alzheimer's disease	26–86
Vascular dementia	28–60
Diffuse Lewy body disease	c. 20

Sources: Burns et al. (1990), Byrne et al. (1989), Cummings et al. (1987), Erkinjuntii (1987).

Other types of mental illness, such as schizophrenia and mania, may occasionally mimic dementia or delirium as disordered thinking and abnormal perceptions lead to apparent memory difficulty and other intellectual problems (some elderly schizophrenics have associated CT scan abnormalities (Naguib and Levy, 1987).

Severe anxiety states may be mistaken for delirium and rarely for dementia, because the high state of arousal may be associated with marked autonomic features, such patients may not be able to respond to questions accurately but can indicate in non-verbal ways that they are aware and orientated. Very rarely individuals with personality disorders may give the appearance of being demented because of a marked degree of self-neglect. These are cases of the Diogenes syndrome, socially isolated, life-long eccentric individuals who often live in self-imposed squalor. Their houses resemble those of the dementia sufferer but they themselves are not cognitively impaired and the condition may be the affects of ageing on 'schizoid' personality.

Organic hallucinosis

Hallucinations in any modality, but most commonly auditory or visual can occur as an isolated psychotic phenomenon not associated with cognitive, behavioural or affective symptoms. The term 'organic' is included as the mechanism is presumed to be due to a physical cause. Visual hallucinations of this type have been attributed to sense organ damage and are sometimes called the Charles Bonnet syndrome (Fuchs and Lauter, 1992). Auditory hallucinations of this type can occur in the alcohol dependence syndrome.

Korsakoff's syndrome (dysmnesic syndrome)

Other brain syndromes such as Korsakoff's syndrome, organic personality change and focal syndromes, such as dysphasia, may sometimes be mistaken for dementia. None of these conditions are associated with marked impairment of intellectual function.

In Korsakoff's syndrome the main deficit is impairment of recent memory while intelligence and personality are relatively well preserved. Korsakoff's syndrome may be caused by anoxia, but most commonly occurs in conditions which lead to Vitamin B_1 deficiency – alcoholism and carcinoma of the stomach. Korsakoff's syndrome, due to alcohol abuse, is amenable to treatment and with abstinence may slightly improve, acute onset having a better prognosis.

Organic personality change

Occurs when the brain (usually in frontal areas) has been damaged by such factors as trauma, infection, haemorrhage. The major deficit is an alteration in the patient's habitual mode of behaviour and in his or her relationships with others. Subtle defects in intellectual function may be present in some patients, but the personality change is disproportional to these other deficits.

Dysphasia

Dysphasia may give the impression of loss of intellectual capacity. If one observes the non-verbal behaviour of these patients it becomes apparent that they show a normal range of emotion, are orientated and are capable of responding appropriately to their environment.

Transient global amnesia

Transient global amnesia is characterized by a sudden onset of severe impairment of all aspects of memory (personal identity is maintained), with relative preservation of other cognitive abilities and alertness. Attacks usually last only a few hours followed by restoration of normal memory function. During the attack patients are often somewhat bewildered and frequently ask for information, they may be anxious. It occurs from the sixth decade onwards and is not uncommon. Males are more commonly affected than are females. The cause is unknown but recent work suggests a close link with migraine and, in a small minority, with epilepsy (Hodges and Warlow, 1990).

References

Blazer, D., Hughes, D.C, and George, L.K. (1987). The epidemiology of depression in an elderly community population. *The Gerontologist*. **27**: 281–287.

Burns A., Jacoby, R., and Levy, R. (1990). Psychiatric phenomena in Alzheimer's disease III: Disorders of mood. *British Journal of Psychiatry*. **157**: 81–85.

Byrne, E.J., Lennox, G., Lowe, J., and Godwin-Austen, R.B. (1989). Diffuse Lewy body disease: clinical features in 15 cases. *Journal of Neurology, Neurosurgery and Psychiatry* **52**: 709–717.

Cohen-Cole, S.A., and Stoudemire, A. (1987). Major depression and physical illness: special considerations in diagnosis and biologic treatment. *Psychiatric Clinics of North America*. **10**: 1–17.

Crook, T.H. 3d (1990). Assessment of drug efficiency in age-associated memory impairment. *Advances in Neurology* **51**: 211–216.

Cummings, J.L., Miller, B., Hill, M.A., and Neshkes, R. (1987). Neuropsychiatric aspects of multi-infarct dementia and dementia of the Alzheimer type. *Archives of Neurology*. **44**: 389–393.

Erkinjuntti, T. (1987). Types of multi-infarct dementia. *Acta Neurologica Scandenavica*. **75**: 391–399.

Fuchs, T., and Lauter, H. (1992). Charles Bonnett syndrome and musical hallucinations in the elderly. In *Delusions and Hallucinations in Old Age*. Katona, C. and Levy, R. (eds). London: Gaskell.

Gilhome, K., Herbst, K. and Humphrey, C. (1980). Hearing impairment and mental state in the elderly living at home. *British Medical Journal*. **281**: 903–905.

Hodges, J.R. and Warlow, C.P. (1990). The aetiology of transient global amnesia. A case control study of 114 cases with prospective follow-up. *Brain*. **113**: 639–657.

Hultsch, D.F., Hammer, M., and Small, B.J. (1993). Age differences in cognitive performance in later life: Relationships to self-reported health and active life style. *Journal of Gerontology*. **48**: 1–11.

Kiloh, L.G. (1961). Pseudodementia. *Acta Psychiatrica Scandinavia*. **37**: 336–351.

Morgan, K., Dallosso, H.M., Arie, T., Byrne, E.J., Jones, R., and Waites, J. (1987). Mental health and psychological well-being along the old and the very old at home. *British Journal of Psychiatry*. **150**: 801–807.

Naquib, M. and Levy, R. (1987). Late paraphrenia – neuropsychological impairment and structural brain abnormalities on computed tomography. *International Journal of Geriatric Psychiatry*. **2**: 83–90.

Scheibel, M.E., and Scheibel, A.B. (1978). The dendritic structure of the leimon betz cell. In: *Architectonics of the Cerebral Cortex*. Brazer, M.A.B. and Petsche, H. (eds). New York: Raven, pp. 43–57.

Wells, C.E. (1979). Pseudodementia. *American Journal of Psychiatry*. **136**: 895–900.

Woods, R. and Britton, P.G. (1985). *Clinical Psychology with the Elderly*. London: Croom Helm.

Chapter 5 _____

History and examination of an old person with a confusional state

A favourite vade mecum (Naish and Read, 1966) contains a chapter on the unconscious patient which begins, 'When you are confronted for the first time with an unconscious patient your mind may be as blank as the patient's'. The same appears to be true for confusional states, but the following simple schema should remove the incipient helplessness.

History

Gaining information

In most cases the history cannot be obtained from the patient, either because there is clouding of consciousness or deficits in recent memory. A typical scenario is the old person who is admitted to an Accident and Emergency (A & E) department with no information.

A woman of 89 was referred to A&E by the general practitioner deputizing service. The note which accompanied her read:

> *Dear Doctor,*
>   *? chest.*
>   *Yours etc*

She was mumbling incoherently and only intermittently responded to the interviewer. The Casualty Officer referred her to the on-call geriatric registrar, who immediately reached for one of the essential diagnostic instruments of the geriatrician, the telephone. He (eventually) made contact with the referring deputizing GP who was able to give him the telephone number of the patient's good neighbour who had called the GP in the first place. From her he obtained a clear history of recent events and the name of the patient's only relative who lived in another part of the country.

It is of course, not always so simple to gain information in such circumstances, but too often no attempt is made. If one remembers that very few people exist whose lives touch no-one at all, a spot of imagination and a good deal of persistence can pay dividends. One advantage to home assessment over hospital based assessment is that such sources of information are often to hand, for example the neighbour who pops her head out of the window as you pass or the note from a district nurse seen on the kitchen table.

What to ask

The history of a confusional state contains the same elements as are found in examples of good history taking practice in younger people – the history of the presenting complaint, the nature of the presenting complaint, past medical and past psychiatric history, family history. Management of an elderly person with a confusional state is often crucially influenced by the social circumstances of the patient and a social history is vital in all cases.

Three simple questions will elicit some fundamental information and thus provide a basis for syndrome diagnosis and immediate management:

How and when did it start?

How did it progress?

How has their physical health been?

A flow chart which shows the syndrome diagnoses suggested by responses to these questions is shown in Fig. 5.1. In this figure, the more likely syndrome is placed first in each box. For example, if the onset is sudden, both delirium and depression are more likely than dementia. Some questions need amplification, for example if the progress was fluctuating, try to establish the nature of the fluctuation; if the condition fluctuates within a day, being worse in the morning it suggests depression, whereas being worse in the evening suggests delirium; if the condition fluctuates from day to day or from week to week it is more likely to be dementia, although sub-acute delirium is also possible. With a combination of responses to these simple questions, a likely syndrome diagnosis will emerge. It should be noted however, that the syndromes are not mutually exclusive, delirium, sub-acute delirium and depression

Table 5.1 Social factors in the history of a confusional state in an old person.

Personal support	Accommodation, type, shared or alone, ownership.
	Help in the home? – from whom
	Help in the home? – of what type
	People to turn to for help?
	Family local? Day Centre/hospital?
Psychological support	Family?) In whom they can confide
	Friends?)
Financial support	Income support?
	Council tax relief?
	Attendance allowance?

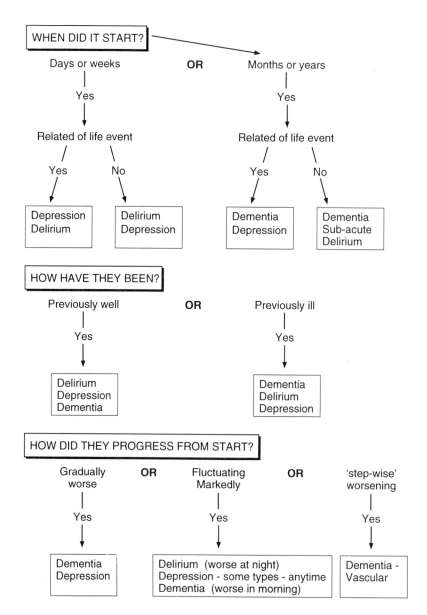

Fig. 5.1 Likely syndrome diagnosis by three simple questions about cognitive impairment.

are frequently superimposed on dementia and because depression in old people is commonly associated with physical illness it may occur with delirium. The answer to the question, 'how have they been', will often clarify the mutual existence of two syndromes.

History-taking is also used to tease out possible aetiological factors.

Important points to ask about the history of the individuals previous health (apart from a list of past illnesses) are; alcohol use, recent trauma, falls, incontinence, smoking and drug use both prescribed and non-prescribed (over the counter medication). In establishing the family history, ask about age and cause of death of family members and ask specifically for family history of hypertension, stroke, dementia, depression, movement disorder. Social factors of importance can be grouped under three headings: *personal support, psychological support, financial support*. Table 5.1 lists under each heading the factors to be considered.

Examination

The traditional mode of examination, whether of mental status or of physical status – look, listen, feel – still applies even where the patient is unable to understand questions fully. When first confronted by this situation the student (or even qualified doctors) may be thrown out of carefully inculcated schemes of examination. The important principle to bear in mind is that anything that a patient says or does may be a clinical sign of diagnostic significance.

Look
The examination begins as soon as one first sees the patient. A wealth of information can be observed or inferred before the first question is asked by the examiner. Figure 5.2 shows some of these observations in schematic form.

Listen
While taking a history from a patient many of the important features of the mental status can be examined. Unfortunately, too often when a patient is unable, for one reason or another, to respond to questions no attempt at a mental state examination is made.

> *A 65 year-old man was admitted to a psychiatric ward from A&E. He had been taken to casualty by the police who had found him wandering around a shopping centre in the early hours of the morning. The police had established that he was a homeless person who was known to abuse alcohol. The casualty officer found that he was not intoxicated (a blood alcohol level was negative).*

In the history notes were the following comments 'poor historian says he had some hassle'. The examination notes read 'No abnormal clinical signs – poor memory ?Korsakoff's'. The psychiatrist's examination of his mental state included the following 'looks perplexed, slightly fatuous in his manner, slow speech . . . unable to give a history because of recent memory problems . . . probable Korsakoff's? Wernickes'. Later that morning he was seen by the consultant. Nurses on the ward reported that he had been restless all night, wandering around the ward and rubbing his head, he repeatedly said that he had 'had some hassle'. He was also reported to be variable in his 'confusion'. The consultant's notes of examination included the following, 'looks perplexed, drifts in and out of awareness, slow speech with marked

LOOK AT THE PATIENT

STROKE

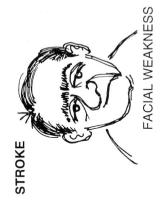

FACIAL WEAKNESS

ANXIETY

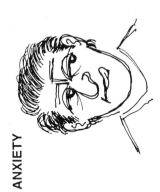

DRY MOUTH
LICKING LIPS

DEPRESSION

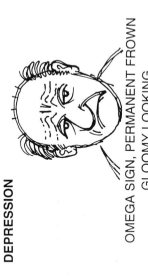

OMEGA SIGN, PERMANENT FROWN
GLOOMY LOOKING

THYROTOXICOSIS

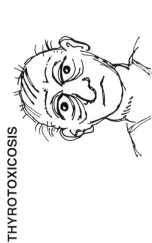

STARING EYES, OEDEMA, MYXOEDEMA
THIN HAIR AND EYEBROWS
DRY SKIN, GOITRE

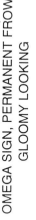

Fig. 5.2   Examination observations

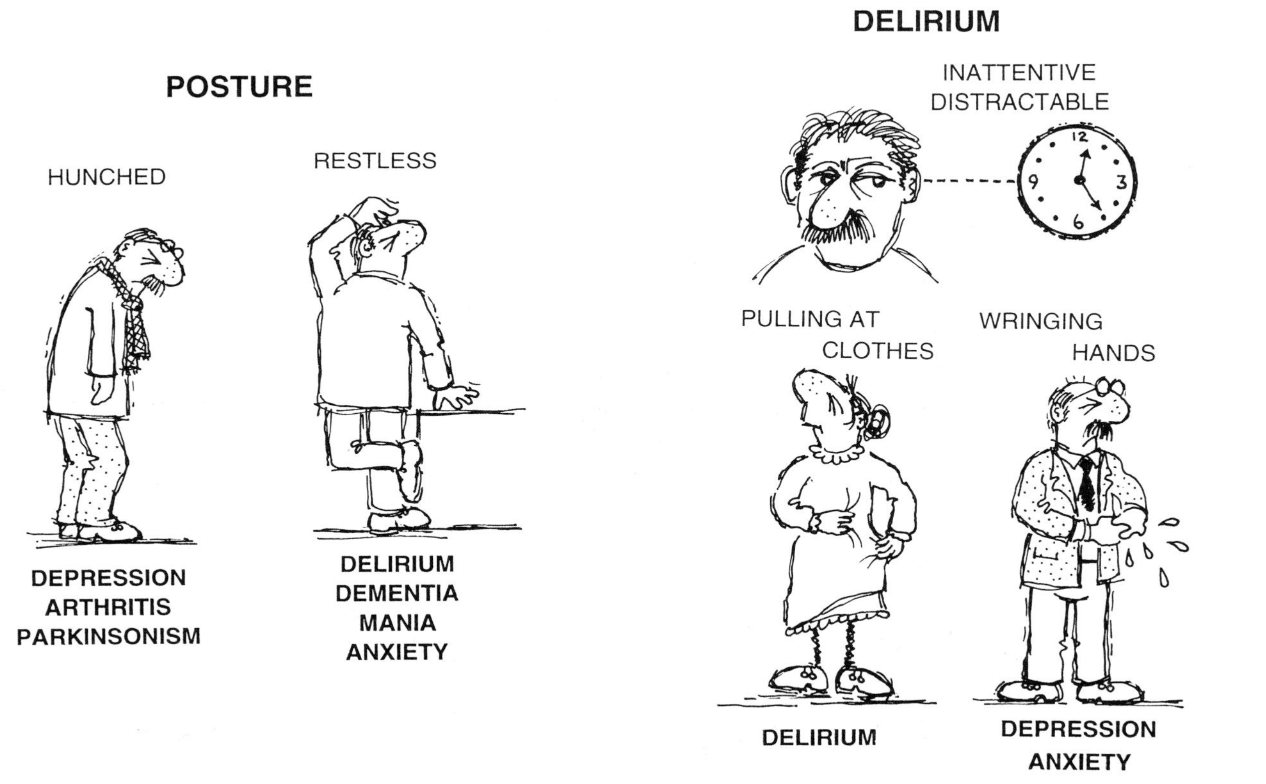

DELIRIUM

INATTENTIVE
DISTRACTABLE

PULLING AT
CLOTHES

WRINGING
HANDS

DELIRIUM

DEPRESSION
ANXIETY

POSTURE

HUNCHED

RESTLESS

DEPRESSION
ARTHRITIS
PARKINSONISM

DELIRIUM
DEMENTIA
MANIA
ANXIETY

Fig. 5.2 (continued)

GAIT AND MOVEMENT

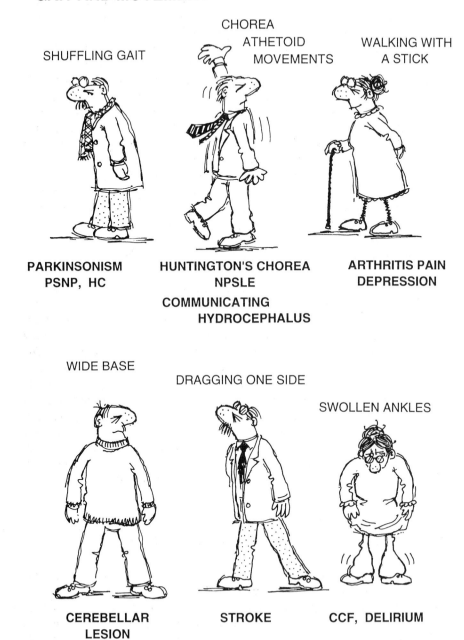

Fig. 5.2 (continued)

perseveration, no dysphasia, appears to be in pain . . . marked attentional deficit and poor immediate registration'. On physical examination the consultant noted bruising to the left shoulder and torso and a haematoma on the left frontal area of the skull was palpated.

This patient made a good recovery after the evacuation of bilateral frontal haematomas which he had incurred as the consequence of a fight in a pub, during which he had fallen and hit his head on the corner of the fireplace. On admission he was suffering from a sub-acute confusional state with marked frontal lobe features – fatuous affect, slowness of cognition and perseveration. He was also repeatedly telling his examiners that he had 'had some hassle', when he was asked directly what he meant by that he was able to say, albeit later in the interview as an unrelated response, 'I was fighting'.

In this case a conversational model of mental status examination was used by the consultant. This essentially comprises throwing away the formal structure of the traditional mental status examination and, in the course of having a 'chat' with the patient, examining each of the features contained in the more formal structure.

For example, the 'listening' part of examination begins when the doctor greets the patient and introduces themselves. The nature of the interchange and the type of response that the patient gives touches on a number of cognitive functions and affective responses. The cognitive aspects of giving a socially appropriate greeting are; attention, registration, comprehension, language, speech, memory, frontal inhibition of socially inappropriate behaviour and frontal sub-cortical control of the speed of response. The affective aspects which may be observed in the nature of the greeting are; anxiety (restlessness, autonomic over-arousal), depression (hunched posture, gloomy expression, slow response, sighs), elation (restless or over-active, jovial or irritable, over-familiar). Other possible responses are; suspiciousness, avoidance, aggression, perplexity, preoccupation and a normal greeting. This simple exercise demonstrates an important part of the clinical examination, the qualitative aspects of assessment. How a patient approaches a task is often more revealing than the quantitative results.

Formal assessment of mental status

The more formal assessment of mental status, especially tests of cognitive function must be placed in the context of the examination as a whole; someone who is behaviourally depressed may well score badly on formal tests but to interpret this as permanent cognitive failure is inappropriate. A useful maxim is when in doubt repeat the test. Even if there is little doubt repeated testing in the assessment of cognitive function in confusional states is very useful because of the fluctuation which characterizes many of them.

Assessment of mental status should include not only a search for deficits but also a search for abilities. Two individuals may have the same poor score on quantitative estimation of cognition yet one is able to safely live independently and the other will require round-the-clock care (Arie 1973). The former is only just out in their responses and demonstrates a grasp of their current situation, the latter is wildly inaccurate and believes that 'my mother will look after me'.

The final introductory comment is that *there are no tests for dementia*. There are no short cuts to a proper assessment, cognitive tests are screening not diagnostic instruments. Examples of brief cognitive screening tests are the mini mental states examination (MMSE – Folstein et al., 1975) the mental states questionnaire (MSQ – Kahn et al. 1960) and the Clifton Assessment procedure for the elderly (CAPE – Pattie and Gilleard, 1975).

Non-cognitive features

The important non-cognitive features are summarized in Table 5.2. Each sign is followed by a list of the confusional states in which it may occur or an indication of the probable site of the lesion. The assessment of mood is of particular importance. There are a number of standardized tests designed for use with old people, such as the Geriatric Depression scale (GDS –Sheik and Yesavage, 1986), the Brief Assessment Schedule Depression Cards (BASDEC – Adshead et al., 1992), and the Hospital Depression and Anxiety scale HAD – Zigmond and Snaith, 1983).

Psychotic features in confusional state are sometimes apparent, but often direct questions have to be posed. To elicit delusions a question such as 'Have you had any unusual experiences recently?' can be posed. To elicit hallucinations, the question 'Have you ever heard or seen things which others have not noticed?' can be used.

Examination of cognition

Table 5.3. shows those aspects of cognitive function which should be assessed in the examination of the old person with a confusional state. Examination of orientation, memory, language concentration and visuo-spatial function are usually included in brief standardized tests of cognitive function such as the mini mental state examination (MMSE – Folstein et al. 1975). Few of the brief standard tests adequately assess frontal lobe function and most do not fully assess praxis or gnosis. It should be again noted that none of the brief tests of cognitive function provide a complete examination of cognitive function nor do they allow credit to the patient for almost accurate answers (the exception here is the 'Newcastle dementia scale – Roth and Hopkins 1953). They may, however, provide a useful framework for examination. The following discussion is not comprehensive and is intended to make a few general points.

Table 5.2 Examination of mental state in confusional states.

Symptom	Possible syndrome or site of lesion
Appearance	Look for features as in Fig. 5.2
Speech	
Rate	Slow: depression, frontal-subcortical lesions
	Fast: mania, dis-inhibition
	Staccato: cerebellar lesions
	Explosive: pseudo-bulbar palsy
Volume	Reduced: thalamic or striatal lesions, depression, personality disorder
Form	Little spontaneous: depression, non-fluent dysphasia
	Syntax errors but spontaneous: fluent dysphasia, low intelligence
	Garbled: jargon aphasia, word salad, formal thought disorder (schizophrenia), delirium, mania
Content	Depressed: 'Oh dear', 'I'm finished' numerous 'Don't know' responses, pessimism, nihilism
	Persistent themes: perseveration (frontal lesions), delusional ideas
	Grandiose: mania
	Paranoid: paranoid state, dementia, mania
Mood	
Depression	May occur in all causes of confusional state
Anxiety	May occur in all causes of confusional state
Mania	Dementia, delirium
Perceptions	
Delusions	Paranoid: dementia, depression, schizophrenia, mania, delirium
	Grandiose: mania
	Nihilistic: depression
	Guilt: depression
Hallucinations	Visual: dementia, delirium, schizophrenia
	Auditory: dementia, delirium, sensory, schizophrenia
Misidentifications:	Dementia, delirium, sensory impairment
Illusions	Delirium, dementia, sensory impairment

Table 5.3 Cognitive features to be examined in old people with confusional states

Orientation, time, place, person
Memory, recent, remote
Attention and concentration
Grasp and judgement
Calculation
Praxis, gnosis
Visuospatial function
Language

Orientation

Orientation is assessed for time (day, date, time of day, and so on), place and person as this is the sequence of loss in cognitive disorders. It is useful always to write down the patient's exact responses for all questions. This not only provides a 'baseline' for comparison with future tests, but also allows an assessment of ability. For example, a person who is only 2 days out on the day of the week and one month out on the month has a higher level of orientation than someone who is 5 days out on the day and 6 months out on the month. Try to establish whether the patient can use 'cues', for example if a 'don't know' response is obtained for the year, give them a list of years to chose from. This not only provides an estimate based on the ability to respond to 'cues', but also gives the patients who may be aware of 'failing' the test a chance to succeed which increases the chances of the test being completed.

Memory

Ask yourself this question: what was I doing on this day 6 months ago? Don't be surprised if it is a bit of a struggle to recall, this is normal! Memory decays over time, yet we expect an old person, who may have lived for nearly a century, to be able to recall all the places where they have lived and worked in the correct sequence. In testing memory one is also able to get an idea of the patient's grasp and judgement. They may recall that they wandered yet be unperturbed by the fact that it was onto a busy road in the middle of winter.

Attention and concentration

If the examiner has not reached a conclusion about the patient's ability to attend by the time the history-taking is concluded, he or she is unlikely to do so on the basis of a test like the serial 7s. The time allowed for this test is 2 minutes and the patient is allowed 3 errors. The serial 7s test is useful as an indication of perseveration as in the following sequence, 93, 86, 93, 93, 93. It may also be helpful in quantifying the degree of cognitive slowing, which is most apparent in frontal sub-cortical lesions or in severe depression.

Grasp and judgement

There are few formal tests for these abilities yet they have important implications for management. The 80 year-old whose reality comprises of living in their childhood home with their mother and who is unconcerned by the fact that the electricity has been cut off because of a failure to regulate their financial affairs, is severely compromised in their ability to live independently. On the other hand, someone who knows (most of the time) that they are failing cognitively and who sticks notes up at home to remind themselves of appointments, is likely to be able to continue to determine their own future.

These abilities are inferred from the history and examination and are only completely assessed with the addition of information from collateral sources.

Visuospatial function

An extremely useful clinical test, which assesses many aspects of cognitive function including visuo-spatial function, is the clock drawing test. This consists of asking the patient to 'draw a clock' on a sheet of paper with a circle drawn on it. When they have completed the task, ask them to put in the hands (if they have not already done so) to indicate a standard time. This test is not only 'user friendly' but is also quick and easy to repeat. It has been validated as a test of cognitive function against standard instruments such as the MMSE (Shulman et al. 1986) and simple scoring schemes have been devised (Shulman et al 1986; Wolf-Klein et al., 1989). It has also been evaluated on a busy medical ward (Huntzinger et al., 1992) and found to be a useful screening test for cognitive impairment in that situation. It is especially useful to quantify deficits over time as in acute or sub-acute confusional states. Examples of this are shown in the chapters 6 and 8. There is no reason why 'b.d' clocks should not be ordered as routinely as 'b.d' blood pressure recordings.

As with all tests of cognition the clock drawing test can be used to assess the qualitative aspects of examination. How does the patient approach the task – the depressed person may stare at the paper and slowly complete it with many requests for reassurance of their competence, whereas the person with dementia may rapidly complete an incorrect clock and appear unaware of their errors. A note should also be made of what the patient says as they perform the test, how long it takes them to complete it (if at all) and their response to the task.

Examination of physical status

A complete examination of physical status should be performed in all patients with confusional states. You are looking for conditions which may be aetiological, for example signs of a stroke in a patient with an acute confusional state and for conditions which may aggravate pre-existing cognitive impairment, such as constipation in the patient with the dementia syndrome. Negative findings are as important as positive findings, the patient with an apparent acute confusional state with no abnormality demonstrable on examination may be suffering from depression rather than delirium. On the other hand, do not ignore positive findings as with the bruising in the patient described earlier in this chapter.

Neurological examination is of particular importance not only to detect 'focal' signs but also to detect release phenomena or premature reflexes which are more common in dementia (especially in Alzheimer's disease). A useful description on the neurological examination in elderly people is given in Godwin-Austen and Bendall, 1990 and of the neurological examination in dementia (including a comprehensive review of the elicitation of premature reflexes) in Paulson, 1971.

Summary

1. Make every effort to obtain a history especially of the onset and progression of the condition.
2. Start your examination of mental state as soon as you meet the patient.
3. Conversation is a useful examination.
4. Standard tests of cognition are screening instruments and can be used as a framework for examination.
5. Test for ability as well as for deficit.
6. Qualitative observations are useful clinical signs.

References

Adshead, F., Cody, D.D., Pitt, B. (1992). BASDEC: a novel screening instrument for depression in the elderly. *British Medical Journal.* **305**: 397.

Arie T. (1973). Dementia in the elderly: management. *British Medical Journal.* **ii**: 602–604

Folstein, M.F., Folstein, J.E., McHugh, P.R. (1975). Mini-mental state: a practical method for grading the cognitive state of patients for the clinician. *Journal of Psychiatric Research.* **12**: 189–198.

Godwin-Austen, R. and Bendall, J. (1990). The neurological examination of the elderly patient. In *The Neurology of the Elderly. London: Springer-Verlay, pp. 1–11.*

Huntzinger, J.A., Rosse, R.B., Schwartz, B.L., Ross, L.A. and Deutsch, S.I. (1992). Clock drawing in the screening assessment of cognitive impairment in an ambulatory care setting: a preliminary report. *General Hospital Psychiatry.* **14**: 142–144.

Kahn, R.L., Goldberg, A.I., Pollock, M.and Peak, A. (1960). Brief objective measures for the determination of mental states in the elderly. *American Journal of Psychiatry.* **107**: 326–328.

Naish J. M, and Read A.E.A. (1966). *The Clinical Apprentice: a Hand Book of Bedside Methods. Bristol: John Wright*

Pattie, A.H., Gilleard, C.J. (1975). A brief psychogeriatric assessment schedule: Validation against psychiatric diagnosis and discharge from hospital. *British Journal of Psychiatry.* **127**: 489–493.

Paulson, G.W. (1971). The neurological examination in dementia. *Contemporary Neurology.* **9**: 13–33.

Roth M. and Hopkins B. (1953). Psychological test performance in patients over 60 I: senile psychosis and the affective disorders of old age. *Journal of Mental Science* **79**: 439–450

Sheik, J.I. and Yesavage, J.A. (1986). Geriatric depression scale (GDS): Recent evidence and development of a shorter version. In *Clinical Gerontology: A guide to Assessment and Intervention.* New York: The Haworth Press, pp. 165–173.

Shulman, K.I., Shedletsky, R. and Silver, I.L. (1986). The challenge of time: clock drawing and cognitive function in the elderly. *International Journal of Geriatric Psychiatry*. **1**: 135–140.

Wolf-Klein, G.P., Silverstone, F.A., Levy, A.P. and Brod, M.A. (1988). Screening for Alzheimer's disease by clock drawing. *Journal of the American Geriatric Society*. **37**: 730–734.

Zigmond, A.S. and Snaith, R.P. (1983). The hospital anxiety and depression scale. *Acta Psychiatria Scandinavia* **67**: 361–370.

Chapter 6 _____

Confusional states with acute onset and rapid course

The mode of onset of the confusional states, as has previously been discussed (Chapter 5), provides a reasonable guide to the syndrome diagnosis. As a general rule, most causes of the dementia syndrome have an onset over many months or years, whereas delirium has an onset over hours or days (sub-acute delirium may be days or a week or so). Acute onset in this chapter refers to very brief time periods, hours or a few days. The course of such states in old people is not well documented but few last more than one month.* The exception in this chapter, is the rare instance where dementia may have a very rapid onset but where its course is variable, very short (months) or long (years).

The knowledge of the prevalence of disease is an aid to diagnosis, one needs to be aware of 'canaries' but diagnosis is more often a 'sparrow' (see Chapter 1). Table 6.1 lists the commonest causes of acute confusional states in old people – the 'sparrows', and Table 6.2 is a comprehensive list of causes which includes a fair number of 'canaries'.

Table 6.1 The commonest causes of acute confusional state in old people

Very common	
Heart failure	Left ventricular failure, Congestive cardiac failure
Infection	Urinary
	Respiratory
Carcinomatosis	
Common	
Cerebrovascular	Transient ischaemia, Drugs
Drugs	Anticholinergic (e.g. tricyclic antidepressants, benzhexol)
	Interactions
	Withdrawal (alcohol, benzodiazepines)
Metabolic	Hypoglycaemia
	Disorders of fluid and electrolyte balance
	Renal or hepatic failure
Anoxia	Respiratory, anaemia, reduced cerebral perfusion

Source: Royal College of Physicians (1981), Lipowski (1992).

_____

*DSM-IIIR criteria for delirium make no stipulation about duration, however, in the notes relating to the criteria they state: 'The duration of an episode of delirium is usually brief, about one week; it is rare for delirium to persist for more than a month'. The duration in the literature is much longer see Chapter 7.

Table 6.2 Causes of delirium (acute or sub-acute) in old people (aged 65 years or more)

Central nervous system		
Cerebrovascular	Stroke, (infarction embolus hypertension) Transient cerebral ischaemia	
(post-traumatic)	Sub-dural haematoma Extra-dural haemorrhage Venous Thrombosis Sub-araconoid haemorrhage cerebrovascular -sludge syndrome Orthostatic hypotension hypertension (Encephalopathy) Cerebral aneurism (haemorrhage or size) Intra vascular coagulation Neoplasm	
Cerebral tumour	Primary – astrocytoma meningioma Secondary – metasteses, primary lung, breast, colon, melanoma	
Infection	Neurosyphilis, brain abscess,	
– intracranial	tuberculosis, meningo-encephalitis Whipple's disease, septic emboli AIDS	
– extracranial	Respiratory, urinary, influenza, septicaemia, sub-acute-bacterial endocarditis, malaria, typhoid, typhus, trypanosomiasis, pancreatitis	
Trauma	Concussion, haemorrhage, communicating hydrocephalus, burns, fat embolus, multiple injuries	
Epilepsy	Ictal, post-ictal	
Auto-immune	Neuropsychiatric systemic lupus erythematosus (NPSLE), Rheumatoid-(nodule, arteritis). Sarcoidosis	

Cardiovascular disease
Myocardial infarction, heart failure (right or left sided), arrhythmia,   aortic stenosis, hypovolemia

Metabolic disorders	
Organ failure	Liver, kidney, lung
Electrolyte disorders	K^+, $Ca^\#$, $Mg^\#$, Na^+,
Water balance	Inappropriate secretion of antidiuretic hormone dehydration, water intoxication
Acidosis	Diabetes mellitus, renal, pulmonary, diarrhoea
Alkalosis	Pulmonary, hyperadrenal-corticism
Deficiency states	Vitamins – B_{12}, thiamine nicotinic acid folate iron, hypoproteinaemia
Endocrine disorders	Hypo- and hyper-thyroidism, Hypo and hyper parathyroidism, diabetes mellitus, Addison's disease, Cushing's disease, hypopituitrism
Miscellaneous	
Toxins	Lead, arsenic, organic mercury, carbon disulphide, insecticides, pesticides, carbon monoxide, alcohol and drugs (including withdrawal states) plants (fungi)
Temperature regulation	Hypothermia, heat stroke, febrile illness

Environment   Radiation exposure, electric shock
Others
  Serum sickness, pernicious anaemia, gall-stones, hyperviscosity (leukaemia,
  polycythemia) porphyria, solvent-sniffing, sickle-cell disease, carcinoid
  syndrome, hyperlipidaemia.

Sources: Beresin (1988), Liston (1982), Lindesay et al., (1990), Lishman (1987), Kim
(1980), Heilman and Fisher (1974), Cairncross and Posner (1984), Ramrakha and
Barton (1993).

Delirium

> An 88 year old widow who lived in warden-aided accommodation presented with
> an acute confusional state.
>   Previously independent, over the course of one weekend, she began to wander
> from her home, phone her daughter requesting information as to the time of
> day and complained of thirst. On admission she was found to have a urinary
> tract infection. Treatment of this did not resolve her confusional state. Further
> investigations revealed primary hyperparathyroidism which was successfully
> treated surgically (Byrne et al., 1987).

In this case, a good history of a rapid onset in a previous cognitively intact
woman was available. Examination confirmed the presence of an acute
confusional state, she was distractible and restless and was worse at night. Her
cognition was not improved (after more than a week) by treating the obvious
and common cause of her confusional state, the urinary tract infection. She
was less floridly ill at this state and was sub-acutely delirious. The important
point here is that she should have recovered quickly if the urinary tract
infection was the sole cause of her problems. In a patient with a pre-morbidly
intact brain, this seems to be the case but if she had had a pre-existing dementia
syndrome or less than perfect cognitive function one would have allowed
considerably longer for expected recovery period – 6 to 8 weeks.

A second contributing factor was then sought (it should perhaps have been
sought on admission) and eventually surgical treatment was successful. As in
many cases where old people are referred for surgery, the surgeon needed
to be reassured of the aetiological significance of the hypercalcaemia to her
cognitive state and her fitness for surgery. The former was demonstrated
by longitudinally correlating her cognitive and functional abilities with the
corrected serum calcium levels. The usefulness of the clock drawing test in this
case, demonstrating changes before and after surgery is shown in Fig. 6.1.

> A 73 year-old man, was referred with a diagnosis of acute senile dementia. For
> one week he had been noted to be forgetful and disorganized in activities of
> everyday living and for 2 nights before admission he had been much worse.
> Systems enquiry did not reveal any abnormality. On examination a large
> pulsatile mass was found in the abdomen. The mass was dull to percussion.
> Despite careful enquiry, neither the patient nor his wife reported any abnormal-
> ity of urinary function. The visiting psychiatrist (with her mind on canaries not

sparrows) referred the patient for surgical admission with a diagnosis of leaking abdominal aneurism. Despite the denial of urinary symptoms his bladder was very grossly enlarged and he was found to have an obstructive encephalopathy.

The floridness of the delirium should have alerted her to the more likely diagnosis, the hypotension or hypovolaemia from an aneurism would be more likely to cause a sub-acute cognitive impairment rather than delirium, in a previously fit 73 year-old with no evidence of cerebrovascular disease. The surgical house officer began a rapid cure by catheterization.

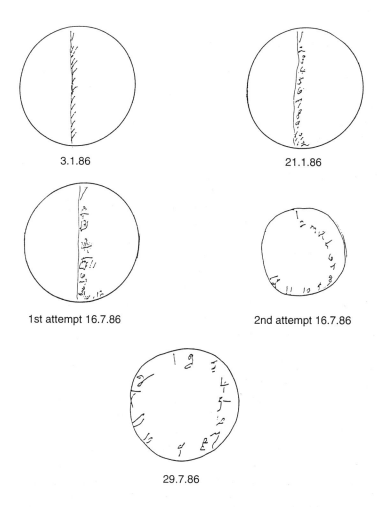

Source: Reproduced with permission from Byrne et al. (1987).

Fig. 6.1 Changes in clock drawing test before and after operation for parathyroidadenoma

Delirium with pre-existing dementia

A 65 year-old divorced woman was admitted for assessment of a deterioration in her 'Alzheimer's disease'. Eleven years previously she had been diagnosed as having Alzheimer's disease and for ten years following this diagnosis had not deteriorated at all. Although divorced she lived in the same house as her ex-husband and reported spending most of her time smoking and listening to the radio. In the two weeks before admission, she had become suddenly immobile with incontinence of urine, and was reported to be more 'confused'. Previous ill-health included empyema (with resultant pneumonectomy), alcohol abuse and gastric ulceration (with gastrectomy).

Although the onset of the presenting episode in this case was very rapid, there was a clear history of long-standing cognitive impairment. However, Alzheimer's disease does not lead to plateaux of stable cognition lasting for 10 years (plateaux of 1 to 2 years have been described, e.g. Katzman, 1985).

The case records of the initial admission 11 years previously were examined and provided a remarkably clear description of a sub-acute delirium. The patient's problems had begun with forgetfulness over a couple of months, then over a period of one week she became much worse with nocturnal exacerbation of her difficulties. The nursing records of her admission confirmed the nocturnal exacerbation. The diagnosis of Alzheimer's disease was made by a neurologist on the basis of a pneumo-encephalogram (her illness began in 1969 before computed tomography was available) which was reported as showing cerebral atrophy.

Examination on admission for the presenting episode confirmed the presence of a delirium. The patient showed an unusual feature, occupational delirium where the patient mimics by gesture the actions of their occupation. Her 'occupation' for 10 years had been smoking, she mimed the action of getting a cigarette out of a packet and matches out of a box, lit the imaginary cigarette and then flicked ash over the doctor.

The diagnosis of the initial episode was felt to be incorrect and she was thought to have had an acute condition leading to dementia which was non-progressive whose aetiology was unclear. Her current episode was thought to be a delirium possibly due to a stroke. A CT scan showed grossly dilated cerebral ventricles with an occluded aqueduct. The diagnosis was then clear; she had communicating hydrocephalus and had probably had it for 11 years. As in this case, the aqueduct may collapse in communicating hydrocephalus.

Following the insertion of an atrio-ventricular shunt her continence and mobility were restored and her delirium resolved, she unfortunately remained demented but was able to return home. This case also demonstrates how diagnosis is so influenced by available knowledge. Hakim and Adams described 'normal pressure' or communicating hydrocephalus in 1965; this patient first presented in 1969 when only a few subsequent cases had been described. There are, however, no mitigating circumstances surrounding the incorrect initial syndrome diagnosis.

Drugs and delirium

Drugs may cause mild or discrete impairment of cognitive function in old people, when they lead to a confusional state this is almost invariably delirium (either acute or, more commonly sub-acute). It is very rare for drugs to be the sole cause of the dementia syndrome (Byrne et al., 1992) they are, however, commonly associated with aggravating already compromised cognitive function. Old people frequently have multiple illnesses leading to poly therapy (Stewart, 1990; Weedle et al., 1990). Some drug interventions are paticularly associated with cognitive impairment, for example, Lithium and Haloperidol (Thomas, 1979).

Table 6.3 gives a more comprehensive list of proprietary drugs known to cause either acute or sub-scute confusional states. Some non-proprietary preparations (over the counter drugs) may also cause acute confusional states, for example, some anti-diarrhoeals contain opiates.

Table 6.3 Drugs causing delirium (acute and sub-acute) in old people

Central nervous system	
Hypnotics and	Benzodiazepines, Barbiturates
Tranquillizers	Phenothiazines, Chloral hydrate
Antidepressants	Tricyclic
	Lithium
	MAOIs
Anticonvulsants	Phenytoin
	Sodium Volproate
	Carbamazepine
Anti-Parkinsonism	Levodopa
	Bromocriptine
	Amantadine
	Orphenadrine
	Benzhexol
	Benztropine
	Procyclidine
Cardiovascular system	
Anti-arrhythmics	Propanolal
	Quinidine
	Procainamide
Antihypertensives	Clonidine
	Methyldopa
	Reserpine
	Diuretics
Cardiac glycosides	Digoxin
Beta blockers	Atenolol
	Propranolol
Nitrates	Isosorbide
Gastrointestinal system	
Anti-diarrhoeals	Atropine
	Hyoscyamine

	Scopolamine
	Homatropine
Anti-nauseants	Cyclizine
Anti-spasmodics	Propantheline
	Methanthelene
Antacids	Cimetidine
	Ranitidine
Anti-obesity	Fenfluramine

Respiratory systems

Antitussives	Opiates
	Synthetic narcotics
Decongestants and	Phenylephrine
Expectorants	Phenylpropanolamine

Musculoskeletal system

Analgesics	Phenacetin
	Salicylates
	Dextropropoxypene
	Opiates
	Synthetic narcotics
Anti-inflammatory	Non-steroidal anti-inflammatory
	drugs (NSAIDS)
	e.g. indomethcin
	Corticosteroids
Muscle relaxants	Diazepam
	Carisoprodol
	Baclofen

Miscellaneous

Anti-histamines	Dyphenhydramine
	Brompheniramine
	Promethazine
	Triprolidine
	Phenindamine
Hypoglycaemics	Insulin
	Oral hypogbycaemics
Anti-malarials	Chloroquine
Alcohol treatment	Disulfiram
	Chlormethiazole
Antibiotics	Penicillins (hypersensitivity reaction)
	Streptomycin
Anti-tuberculous	Osoniazid
	Rifampicin
Anti-neoplastic agents	Corticosteroids
	Procarbazine

Sources: Davison (1981), Lindesay et al. (1990), Lipowski (1992), Liston (1982), Beresin (1988), Lipowski (1990).

References

Beresin, E.V. (1988). Delirium in the elderly. *Journal of Geriatric Psychiatry and Neurology* **1**: 127–143.

Byrne E.J., Hosking D.J. and Jameson, C. (1987). Serial assessment of serum calcium correlates with mental state. *International Journal of Geriatric Psychiatry* **2**: 163–168.

Byrne, E.J., Smith, C.W., Arie, T. and Lilley, J. (1992). Diagnosis if dementia 3 – Use of investigations. A survey of current consultant practice, review of the literature and implications for audit. *International Journal of Geriatric Psychiatry* **7**: 647–657.

Cairncross, J.G., Posner, J.B. (1984). *Brain tumours in the elderly in clinical neurology of Aging*. Albert, M.L. (ed.). Oxford: Oxford University Press pp. 445–457.

Davison, K. (1981). Toxic psychosis. *British Journal of Hospital Medicine*. **26**: 530–537.

Hakim, S., Adams, R.D. (1965). The special clinical problems of symptomatic hydrocephalus with normal cerebro spinal fluid pressure. *Journal of the Neurological Science* **2** 207–327.

Heilman, K.H., Fisher, W.R. (1974). Hyperlipidemic dementia. *Archives of Neurology* **31**: 67–68.

Katzman, R. (1985). Clinical presentation of the cause of Alzheimer's disease: the atypical patient. *Interdisciplinary Topics in Gerontology* **20**: 12–18.

Kim, R.C. (1980). Rheumatoid disease with encephalopathy. *Annals of Neurology* **7**: 86–91.

Lindesay, J., MacDonald, A. and Starke, I. (1990). *Delirium in the Elderly*. Oxford: Oxford Medical Publications, 43–65.

Lipowski, Z.J. (1990). *Delirium: acute Confusional States*. New York: Oxford University Press, pp. 133–134.

Lipowski, Z.J. (1992). Delirium and impaired consciousness In: *Oxford Text Book of Geriatric Medicine*. Evans, J Gri. and Williams, T.F. (eds). Oxford: Oxford University Press, pp. 490–496.

Lishman, W.A. (1987). *Organic Psychiatry*. Blackwell: Oxford, p. 130.

Liston, E.H. (1982). Delirium in the aged. *Psychiatric Clinical of North America* **5**: 49–66.

Ramrakha, P.S. and Barton, I. (1993). Drug smugglers delirium. *British Journal of Psychiatry* **306**: 470–471.

Royal College of Physicians (1981). Organic mental impairment in the elderly. *Journal of the Royal College of Physicians* **15**: 141–167.

Stewart, R.B. (1990). Polypharmacy in the elderly: a fait accompli DICP-*The annals of Pharmacotherapy*. **24**: 321–323.

Thomas, C.J. (1979). Brain damage with Lithium/Haloperidol. *British Journal of Psychiatry*. **134**: 552.

Weedle, P.B., Poston, J.W., Parish, P.A. (1990). Drug prescribing in the residential homes for elderly people in the United Kingdom. *DICP, The Annals of Phamacotherpy* **24**: 533–536.

Chapter 7

Confusional states with relatively rapid onset and course

Confusional states with relatively rapid onset and course (onset over days or a few weeks, course of a few weeks) are, perhaps, even more common in old people than those with acute onset. There is, however, little research data to support that contention. Mori and Yamadori (1987) studied 41 patients with stroke in the territory of the right middle cerebral artery and found that sub-acute delirium was the most common confusional state in these patients, occurring in 25 (61 per cent), whereas acute delirium occurred in only 6 (15 per cent). (These authors use the term acute confusional state (ACS) to describe such patients, but their definition of ACS is that of sub-acute delirium.) The duration of the two types of delirium in these patients is not given but it is notable that the authors report that the confusional state became chronic (still present at 3 months) in 5 patients. In a recent prospective study of 70 psychogeriatric patients who on admission fulfilled DSM-III R criteria for delirium (Koponen and Riekkinen 1993), the acute type (characterized by hyperactivity and florid psychotic symptoms) was commoner than the sub-acute type ('silent type' characterized by hypoactivity and less florid psychotic symptoms), although the prevalence of each type is not given delusions and hallucinations occurred in over 60 per cent of cases. The mean duration of delirium was 19.5 days (standard deviation ± 15.4 days), and Koponen and Riekkinen found no difference in duration between the subtypes of delirium.

Such studies also illustrate another important point about confusional states, that is that the type of confusional state that an individual clinician encounters most commonly may be influenced both by his or her speciality and the location of the clinical encounter.

Koponen and Riekkinen were seeing patients referred to a specialist psychogeriatric service and it might be expected that they would have a preponderance of patients with behavioural and psychotic symptoms-acute rather than sub-acute delirium. There is also evidence that psychiatrists see fewer patients with multi-infarct dementia than do geriatricians, at least from populations of patients who come to post-mortem (Jellinger et al., 1990).

Sub-acute confusional states

In the previous chapter lists of the causes of delirium were given which did not differentiate between those which may cause the acute types and those which may cause the sub-acute types. This is because there is almost no information available which enables one to do so. Davison 1981 has reviewed the literature on drug toxicity and provides lists of drugs which cause 'behavioural toxicity' – defined as drowsiness, insomnia, vivid dreams and nightmares, mild depression, mild excitement, anxiety, irritability, sensitivity to noise, listlessness and restlessness, and delirium, some drugs such as Benzodiazepines may cause both. For the present time, therefore, the cause of both sub-types of delirium must remain the undifferentiated list shown in Chapter 6 (Tables 6.1 and 6.2).

> *An 86 year-old man presented with a one-month history of memory problems. His wife noted that at about the time of the onset of his problems, he had complained of 'indigestion'. Observation on admission revealed a fluctuating level of consciousness but no hallucinations or delusions. Investigation revealed a recent antero-septal myocardial infarction. He recovered fully after a further two weeks.*

This case illustrates another general point about duration of confusional states, in those with previously intact cognitive function and good previous health they are likely to be of shorter duration, whereas those patients with pre-existing cognitive impairment and poor previous health are likely to have prolonged states, and on recovery from the index episode to suffer a further decline in cognition. There is only evidence in the literature to support the last point (Koponen and Riekkinen, 1993), the other contentions are clinical impressions which remains to be tested.

Dementia with relatively rapid onset and course

Relatively rapid onset here refers to a few weeks or months and duration to months or a year or two. There is some overlap here with what I have described as acute onset and rapid course, see Chapter 6. A list of causes of dementia with relatively rapid onset and course is shown in Table 7.1.

> *A 70-year old woman presented with a one month history of problems with recognising people and parts of her body. She was initially thought to have either a cerebral tumour or a stroke, CT scan was however normal. She rapidly developed a full dementia syndrome with positive clinical signs (myoclonus and ataxia) and investigative findings (EEG – initially asymmetrically abnormal then characteristically abnormal triphasic waves). She died six months after the onset of her illness. Post mortem diagnosis was Creutzfeldt–Jacob disease. The onset of the full blown dementia syndrome was very rapid and the progression, for dementia was likewise very swift.*

There are relatively few causes of the dementia syndrome with very rapid onset (days to weeks), they include; transmissible dementias, post-traumatic dementia, dementia following a massive stroke, herpes simplex, encephalitis and other post-infective states and auto-immune diseases which as systemic lupus erythematosus. The duration and progression of rapid or relatively rapid onset dementia depends on the underlying cause.

Table 7.1 Causes of dementia with relatively rapid onset and course.

Degenerative	Diffuse Lewy body disease, Alzheimer's disease (rare)
Vascular	Cerebral infarction andembolus, cerebral aneurism, cerebral vasculitis
Transmissible dementias	Creutzfeldt-Jakob disease, Gerstmann–Straussler syndrome
Infection	Encephalitis (especially herpes simplex), Whipple's disease
Miscellaneous	Severe cerebral trauma (course may be prolonged), neuropsychiatric systemic lupus, rheumatoid, sarcoid, temporal arteritis

Other confusional states which may mimic dementia with relatively rapid onset

Most of the functional psychiatric disorders which mimic dementia have a relatively rapid onset. The exception is personality disorder. The commonest psychiatric disorder to mimic dementia in old people is depression. Age is an important but unexplained determinant of this phenomenon. McHugh and Folstein 1979, showed that in a group of severely depressed patients of equal severity of illness it was only those patients over the age of 60 years who showed abnormalities in cognitive function. Cognitive disorders in depression have been explained because of the psychomotor retardation and sometimes the psychotic phenomena (depressive delusions or hallucinations), which by preoccupying the patient interfere with normal cognition. The findings of McHugh and Folstein, however, suggest that in old people this is not a sufficient explanation and that the ageing process is more important. It is likely, but not proven, that even in old people, it is the severe form of depressive illness (major affective disorder) rather than milder forms of depression (minor affective disorder, dysthymia) which may mimic dementia.

Depression mimicking dementia

> *A 75-year old man was referred because he was 'no longer able to cope'. Over a period of three months he had become apparently forgetful and unable to care for himself (not cooking, shaving or dressing properly). He looked depressed, spoke very slowly and often wrung his hands and said 'I'm Finished' or 'Oh dear'. On*

cognitive testing he scored 15 out of 30 in the MMSE and many responses were recorded as 'I don't know'. His mother had committed suicide at the age of 70 years. He recovered fully after being treated with Amitiptyline; 10 mg t.d.s.

In this case failure to cope with everyday life was the initial symptom of depression. In some old people depressed mood is not immediately apparent indeed some complain of emptiness or absence of emotion rather than of too much sadness or depression (Georgotas, 1983). The qualitative observation of the way he performed on tests of cognition rather than the results themselves were important diagnostically, as was the family history of presumed depression (suicide).

Paranoid state of late onset mimicking dementia

A 90-year old woman presented with a two-month history of lack of self-care, forgetfulness and reduced sociability. She suffered from bilateral deafness and blindness. Her husband (aged 92 years) was finding it difficult to cope and she was admitted to a nursing home for permanent care. In the home she became aggressive towards other residents and was thus referred. Communication really was not possible but interview with the aid of a hearing aid amplification device revealed paranoid delusions, including an assault from a 'gang from the IRA' who were going to 'get her', and normal cognitive function.

The patient responded well to small doses of neuroleptic medication (Thioridazine; 10 mg t.d.s.)

Preoccupation with inner psychic experiences may lead to apparent cognitive dysfunction. Deafness is associated with an increased occurrence of paranoid disorders in old people (Cooper et al., 1974, Naguib and Levy, 1987) the commonest psychiatric disorder associated with deafness is depression. This lady had double sensory impairment and her near blindness was of recent origin. Other clues to her lack of cognitive impairment came from observations by nursing staff who reported that she found her way about the ward very quickly despite her sensory problems, and that she stood near the ward television while a quiz programme was on and answered many of the questions correctly.

Dysphasic patients may appear to be profoundly cognitively impaired because of their communication problems. In these cases observation and examination using non-verbal tests of cognition should reveal the true state of affairs. Patience and time spent in interviewing such patients can also pay dividends – even the most dysphasic patients can make themselves understood and the dysphasia may vary in intensity from day to day, so that at some times they are able to demonstrate grasp, memory of recent events and other abilities which belie first impressions.

References

Cooper, A.F., Kay, D.W.D., Curry, A.R, Garside, R.F and Roth, M. (1974). Hearing loss in paranoid and affective psychoses of the elderly. *Lancet.* ii: 851–861.

Davison, K. (1981). Toxic psychosis. *British Journal of Hospital Medicine.* **26**: 530–537.

Georgotas, A. (1983). Affective disorders in the elderly: diagnostic and research considerations. *Age and Ageing.* **12**: 1–10.

Jelinger, K., Danielczyk, W., Fischer, P. and Gabriel, E. (1990). Clinicopathological analysis of dementia disorders in the elderly. *Journal of Neurological Sciences.* **95**: 239–258.

Koponen, H.J. and Riekkinen, P.J. (1993). A prospective study of delirium in elderly patients admitted to a psychiatric hospital. *Psychological Medicine* **23**: 103–109.

McHugh P.R. and Folstein, M.F. (1979). Psychopathology of dementia. Implications for neuropathology. In *Congenital and Acquired Cognitive Disorders. Katzman, R. (ed) New York: Raven Press, pp. 17–30.*

Mori, E. and Yamadori, A. (1987). Acute confusional state and acute agitated delirium occurrence after infarction in the right middle cerebral artery territory. *Archives of Neurology.* **44**: 1139–1143.

Naguib, M. and Levy, R. (1987). Late paraphrenia – neuropsychological impairment and structural brain abnormalities on computed tomography. *International Journal of Geriatric Psychiatry* **2**: 83–90.

Chapter 8 _____

Confusional states with gradual onset and prolonged course

This type of natural history of a confusional state in an old person (onset over months, course over years) is almost always due to the dementia syndrome of various aetiologies. Very rarely severe depression may have a very gradual onset and prolonged course (especially when resistant to treatment).

The frequency with which each cause of the dementia syndrome occurs is a matter of controversy. Most of the figures quoted in textbooks are derived from the findings of post-mortem studies. Such studies are not a sufficient database on which to base estimates of frequency because, the samples are highly selected and pathological diagnostic criteria vary considerably between studies (Byrne et al., 1991a). Tierney et al., 1988, in a clinico-pathological study of 57 cases, showed that the frequency of the different causes of dementia varied according to the pathological diagnostic criteria which were used, and Ulrich et al. (1986) have reported similar findings. These observations are of no inconsiderable importance, if pathological findings are regarded uncritically as the gold standard for clinical diagnosis and they are unreliable then not only will false assumptions about clinical features, in particular causes of the dementia syndrome, be made but such studies are less than comparable. Despite these caveats it is likely that Alzheimer's disease will be confirmed as the commonest cause of dementia in all age groups and that vascular dementia (multi-infarct dementia) and dementia associated with Parkinsonian features will be among the most common.

Table 8.1 shows the causes of the dementia syndrome with gradual onset and prolonged course.

Alzheimer's disease

Alois Alzheimer described the clinical and pathological features of the disease which bears his name in 1906 (the case report was published in 1907). It was Kraeplin who subsequently first used the eponymous term Alzheimer's disease (AD).

An 86 year-old widow became very agitated following her recent admission to a residential home. She was demanding to go back to the home of her youth, to

Table 8.1   Causes of dementia in old people (age 65 years or more) with gradual onset and prolonged course.

Degenerative	Alzheimer's disease, Pick's disease, Wilson's disease, Huntington's Chorea, progressive supranuclear palsy, diffuse Lewy body disease, dementia of the frontal lobe type, corticobasal de.g.eneration, multi-system atrophies, multiple sclerosis, motor neurone disease, thalamic dementia.
Vascular	Binswanger's disease (subcortical arteriosclerotic encephalopathy) Multiple lacunar infarction Cerebral infarction, embolus
Infections	Neurosyphilis
Space occupying lesions	Primary intracranial tumours meningioma, astrocytoma chronic sub-dural haematoma
Metabolic and endocrine	Uraemia, chronic hepatic encephalopathy, carcinomatosis, hypothyroidism, hypopituitarism, Addison's disease
Miscellaneous	Communicating hydrocephalus, Alcoholic dementia

look after father and mother, and was accusing staff of stealing her possessions. For the previous 3 years she had become gradually less competent in her ability to look after herself. She had decreasing self-care (a formerly fastidious woman, she stopped bathing) and in the last 6 months difficulty in 'finding the right words' and increasing difficulty in recognizing her family and friends. She had been admitted to hospital following a fall and discharged to the residential home. She then developed paranoid ideas, believing the staff were poisoning her food.

A move to new surroundings is one of the most potent precipitants of further decompensation in old people with AD. The paranoid ideas that she was expressing had been present for some time. As a general rule such patients are likely, at least in the initial settling down period, to require the attention of skilled staff (that is, those trained in the care of psychotic patients). Many residential homes have no such staff. A further medical assessment confirmed a clinical diagnosis of AD. She was treated with small doses of neuroleptics but failed to settle in a nursing home due to her assaultative behaviour (she took to hitting passers by with her stick). She was eventually admitted to a psychogeriatric continuing care ward. The assaultative behaviour continued, but in a milder form and she was able to join in the social activities of the ward and to go on holiday with staff.

Aetiology

The cause of Alzheimer's disease is unknown. Some of the theories about its pathogenesis are summarized in Figure 8.1.

Clinical features

The cognitive abnormalities in AD have been reviewed by a number of authors (see Hart and Semple, 1990) and are summarized in Table 8.2.

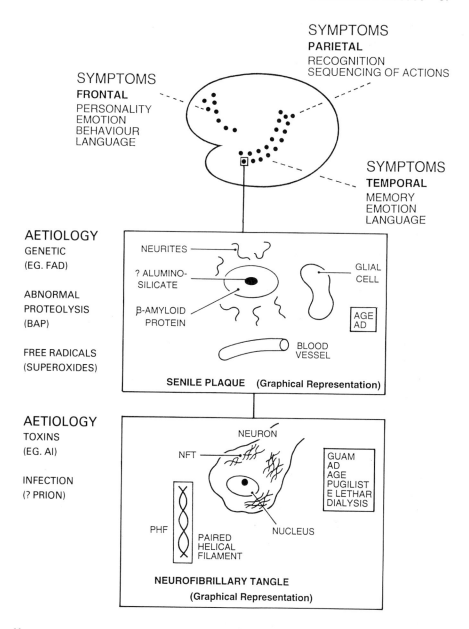

Fig. 8.1 Schematic representation of the possible causes of Alzheimer's disease

Table 8.2 Cognitive function in Alzheimer's disease.

Cognitive function	Deficit	Course
Memory	Central executive component of working memory	
	Temporal disorientation	Early
Personality	Exaggeration of pre-morbid traits	
	Apathy which precludes taking on novel ventures	
	Marked distractibility, especially when fatigued	Early
Visuo-spatial	Spatial disorientation*	
	Constructional disability	Middle
Agnosia	Auditory sound agnosia	
	Astereognosis	Middle
Apraxia	Ideational**	
	Ideomotor	
	'dressing apraxia'	
Language and communication	Naming–nominal aphasia	
	Fluency – speed	
	Fluency – word	
	Comprehension (fluent or expressive dysphasia)	Middle
Intellect	Dyscalculia	
	Grasp	
	Judgement	Middle

*, Spatial disorientation is strongly correlated with impaired memory (Henderson et al., 1989).
**, Ideational apraxia is almost always accompanied by receptive language disturbance (Hart and Semple, 1990)
Source: Hart and Semple (1990), Baddeley et al., (1991), Henderson et al., (1989), Rapcsak et al., (1989), Welsh et al., (1992), Kirk and Kertesz (1991).

One of the most extensive studies of the psychiatric features of AD is that of Burns and colleagues from the Institute of Psychiatry in London. In four papers published in 1990, they described the clinical features under four headings; disorders of thought content, disorders of perception, disorders of mood and disorders of behaviour. Their findings are summarized in Table 8.3.

Course

Most studies give a wide range for duration of AD (from 1 to 20 years or more). The mean survival of AD patients from presentation is about 5–6 years (Heir et al., 1989; Molsa et al., 1986). The course of AD is classically described as a smooth curve of deterioration.

'Atypical' cases, both in clinical features and in course, are documented and are summarized in Table 8.4.

Table 8.3 Psychiatric features of Alzheimer's disease (adapted from Burns et al. 1990a, b, c, d, n = 178).

Disorder	Percentage
Disorders of thought content	
Delusions	15.7%
Persecutory ideation	20.2%
Disorders of perception	
Hallucinations	16.9%
Misidentifications	30.3%
Disorders of mood	
Depression	23.5%
Mania	3.5%
Disorders of behaviour	
Aggression	19.7%
Wandering	18.5%
Sexual disinhibition	6.9%
'Rage'	35.6%
Hypermetamorphosis	31%
Withdrawal/apathy	40.8%

*An excessive tendency to attend and react to every visual stimulus.

Table 8.4 'Atypical' presentations and course in Alzheimer's disease

Presentation	Early language disorders
	Dominant angular gyrus syndrome
	Right parietal syndrome
	Primary visual agnosia
Course	Plateau of stable cognition
	Rapid course

Source: Katzman (1985); Shuttleworth (1984)

Heterogeneity in Alzheimer's disease

Almost from the be.g.inning of the history of AD there has been a debate about sub-types which continues today. This debate has been based on clinical and pathological features in 'young' (often familial cases) and 'old' patients (Roth and Wischik, 1986). It has been suggested that those with an early onset have a more rapid course and a more severe disorder of language than late onset cases (e.g. Chui et al., 1985) and that early onset cases have more widespread and severe pathological changes (Rosser et al., 1984). Recently, the concept of numerous sub-types has been examined (Blennow et al., 1991; Fenn et al., 1993) perhaps the most controversial of which is 'the Lewy body type' of AD (Hansen et al., 1990; Forstal et al., 1993). Until clear and agreed pathological definitions of AD emerge the debate will not be resolved.

Treatment

There is no definitive treatment for AD. Drugs which restore the cholinergic deficiency have been most extensively researched and some (e.g. tacrine) have a modest effect in a small proportion of patients (Eagger et al., 1991). Reviews of the novel agents which have been (or are being) examined include (Byrne and Arie, 1991; Levy, 1991)

Vascular dementia

Because of the increasing evidence for heterogeneity in cases formerly known as multi-infarct dementia (see below) the term vascular dementia is now used in preference.

> *A 76 year-old man was on holiday with his wife and was found by her one night on the fire escape of the hotel. He was disorientated and agitated and said he was looking for the cat.*
>
> *On their return to their home town the following day, he was admitted to a geriatric medical ward. His wife commented that when they had married 6 months previously he was well but in the last few weeks she had noticed that he was a bit forgetful. He had had hypertension treated for 10 years. On examination he was delirious but had no focal neurological signs. Clock drawing during his delirium is shown in Fig. 8.2. CT scan showed a recent infarct in the territory of the right middle cerebral artery with widespread small lacunar infarcts. His confusional state persisted for 12 months and he required continuing care.*

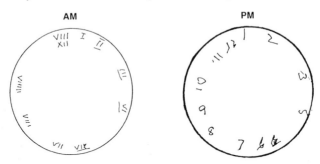

Fig. 8.2   Variability in clock drawing ability in vascular dementia

This man had mild impairment probably due to his lacunar state followed by persistent delirium (as a result of the stroke) resolving to a clear dementia after 12 months. He did not show stepwise progression. He had a clear risk factor in the history of hypertension.

Aetiology

The aetiology of vascular dementia is largely the aetiology of stroke, although a small proportion of cases have other aetiologies, for example neuropsychiatric systemic lupus erythematosus. These other aetiologies are listed in Table 8.5. An extensive review of risk factors for stroke may be found in Ebrahim (1990), in his book on the epidemiology of stroke. Risk factors that have been identified include; hypertension, cigarette smoking, excessive alcohol intake, hyperlipidaemia, heart disease and diabetes mellitus (Meyer et al., 1986; Katona, 1989)

Table 8.5 Causes of vascular dementia

Subarachnoid haemorrhage
Subdural haematoma
Giant cerebral aneurysms
Neuropsychiatric systemic lupus erythematosus
Collagen, vascular disorders
Beurgers disease (thrombo-angiitis obliterons)

Sources: Lishman (1987), Dennis et al., (1992), Chynoweth and Foley (1969).

Heterogeneity of vascular dementia

Vascular dementia may be caused by infarction due to haemorrhage or to thrombosis or to emboli, by the lacunar state and by sub-cortical white matter lesions (demylination, leukoariosis) or by any combination of the three.

Infarction

Large infarcts

Current classificatory systems of vascular lesions (Roman et al., 1993) sub-divide infarction into large, greater than 15 mls of brain tissue and small or lacunes less than 15 mls of brain tissue (often very small 0.5 mls–2 mls).

The classical early studies of Tomlinson et al. (1968, 1970) attributed dementia following infarction to the volume of cerebral tissue that was affected, demented patients having greater than 100 mls of brain infarcted compared to non-demented patients. These studies also pointed out that in non-demented elderly individuals vascular lesions were very common, occurring in 20 of 28 such individuals. Support for both of these observations can be found in more recent literature. Del Ser et al., 1990 found that in cases of pure cerebrovascular disease demented patients had a significantly greater volume of infarction at post-mortem than did non-demented patients, but that greater volume was mostly less than 100 mls. In this study non-demented cases had similar types of lesions but they were less extensive. Mielke et al., (1992) found that the severity of vascular dementia was related to the volume of metabolically impaired tissue estimated in living patients by positron emission tomography (PET).

There is also evidence that dementia can be produced by infarction in certain critical areas of the brain, irrespective of the volume of such infarction. The NINDS-AIREN workshop (Roman et al., 1993) has recently proposed operational diagnostic criteria for vascular dementia (which are controversial) and cite eight such critical areas. The clinical features of thalamic stroke have been reviewed by Katz et al., (1987), and of strokes in mesencephalon and diencephalon by Stienke et al., (1992). Infarction leading to vascular dementia is not always associated with overt stroke (Hershey et al., 1987; Del Ser et al., 1990).

Small infarctions-lacunes

Lacunes are found in areas supplied by small penetrating vessels (when they are occluded) such as basal ganglia, thalamus, internal capsule, optic radiation and pons (Fisher, 1965; Weisberg, 1982). With a few dissenting voices (e.g.; Fisher 1982) the lacunar state (Marie, 1901) is recognized as a sufficient and common cause of vascular dementia (see Delser et al., 1990), which is often associated with hypertension. While the lacunar state usually cause the typical 'step-wise' course of vascular dementia, some cases may have a course similar to that of 'typical' AD, with gradual onset and progression (Weisberg, 1982). Vascular dementia has also been attributed to cortical micro-infarction but this remains controversial.

White matter lesions

Extensive white matter lesions, demylination, in association with dementia were described by Binswanger in 1894, see review by Babikan and Roppan (1987). Such cases are relatively uncommon; however less extensive white matter lesions are found in vascular dementia, AD and in healthy old people. In life they may be detected on CT or NMR scans and Hachinski et al. 1987 have coined the term 'leuko-araiosis' to describe this radiological change. A number of studies have suggested that 'leuko-araiosis' per se is associated with cognitive abnormalities in non-demented individuals (e.g. Steingart et al., 1987) whereas other have not found any such association (e.g. Tupler et al., 1992). A careful pathological study by (Janota et al., 1989) of leuko-araiosis found that extensive confluent peri-ventricular lesions on CT scan were associated with histological changes in white matter, whereas patchy leuko-araiosis was not associated with abnormal histological change.

Clinical features

The clinical features associated with vascular dementia are variable and depend on the location or locations of the lesions. Those features which were found more commonly in demented patients with cerebrovascular disease (compared to non-demented patients) are shown in Table 8.6.

Table 8.6 Clinical features significantly associated with vascular dementia compared to non-demented patients with cerebrovascular disease

Incontinence – urinary, faecal
Pyramidal signs
Gait disturbance

On of the most thorny clinical problems is in distinguishing between dementia due to AD and dementia due to cerebrovascular disease. The most widely used instrument is the Hachinski ischaemia scale (IS – Hachinski et al., 1975), or subsequent variations such as Ettlin et al. 1989. The clinical features which best discriminate between AD and vascular dementia are; focal neurological signs, focal neurological symptoms, history of hypertension, history of strokes and stepwise deterioration (see review by Katona, 1989).

Treatment

There is good evidence that treatment of hypertension in old people reduces the risk of stroke (MRC, 1992). In those with established vascular dementia control of risk factors for stroke can also reduce morbidity. For example Meyer et al. 1986 showed that cognitive function stabilized in such patients if systolic blood pressure was maintained at the high normal range (135–150 mmHg), control of cigarette smoking in the non-hypertensive patients in this study also improved cognition and aspirin showed similar benefit.

Diffuse Lewy body disease (Lewy body variant at Alzheimer's disease, senile dementia of the Lewy body type).

Aetiology

While there is debate about the nosological status of DLB, hence the profusion of names, it is increasingly recognized that DLB is one of the commonest causes of dementia in old people. The name DLB derives from the finding that, in these cases, Lewy bodies are found in both sub-cortical (especially substantia nigra) and cortical (especially cingulate and insular cortex) areas of brain at post-mortem. (e.g. Gibb et al., 1987), some cases show Alzheimer histological change and have therefore been described as a sub-type of Alzheimer's disease (Hansen et al., 1990, Forstal et al., 1993). It is likely that DLB will prove to be a spectrum disorder, with typical Parkinson's disease at one end of the spectrum and 'typical' Alzheimer's disease at the other (Byrne 1991, 1992).

Clinical features

DLB is characterized by dementia in association with Parkinsonism. The dementia is milder at onset than is the case in AD, and visuo-spatial problems are prominent (Hansen et al., 1990, Perry et al., 1990). In addition the cognitive impairment shows marked variability from day to day and within a single day (Williams et al., 1993), and episodes of acute confusional state are frequently observed. Most authors describe the Parkinsonism as mild or not typical of Parkinson's disease, but the larger series show that about a third present with classical Parkinson's disease (e.g. Kosaka, 1990). Psychiatric symptoms are common in some series (Byrne et al., 1989, Perry et al., 1990), especially visual hallucinations, which have been linked to the profound cholinergic deficits in these cases (Perry et al., 1990). Several operational clinical diagnostic criteria have been devised (e.g. McKeith et al., 1993; Byrne et al., 1991a) which should facilitate the study of this condition.

Course

The course of the condition is as variable as its presentation, with a mean duration in the literature of about 5 years. Most cases have a gradual onset and a gradual, albeit fluctuating, course. A few cases have been described with a relatively rapid onset and course, including one woman who was diagnosed as having Creuztfeldt–Jacob disease in life (Byrne et al., 1989).

Treatment

The motor symptoms may be responsive to levadopa (Williams et al., in 1993). Perry et al., (1990) suggest that the cognitive impairment in DLB may respond to anti-cholinergic therapy.

Dementia with Parkinson's disease

A 73 year-old man with Parkinson's disease of 4 years duration was referred to a psychiatrist because he was seeing horses galloping through his front room and little men in his garden. His illness began with a slowness in walking, difficulty in turning over in bed and stooped posture. He was assessed by a neurologist who found, rigidity, hypomimia, festinating gait and postural abnormality, his cognition was described as normal at this time. He made a good initial response to levadopa with carbidopa but over the 4 years his dose was constantly changed as he had episodes of 'confusion' which were attributed to the medication. His wife noticed a gradual decline in his cognitive function-poor memory, disorientation and poor concentration-for the previous 12 months. His treatment had been discontinued 6 months before presentation and he had great difficulty in moving about. The episodes of 'confusion' had persisted during this time. On assessment he had dementia, with marked visuo-spatial disfunction, visual hallucinations and Parkinsonism. Both his motor and his cognitive function varied markedly within a day and from day to day. He was treated with a combination of levadopa and deprenyl in small doses.

His motor symptoms showed a marked improvement and he was more independent. The visual hallucinations persisted as did the episodes of 'confusion' which when observed seemed to be periods of a severe disorder and attention. Small doses of neuroleptics did not improve his hallucinations but did not make his motor symptoms worse.

This man showed 'typical' features of diffuse Lewy body disease, fluctuation in cognition state, visual hallucinations and Parkinsonism. His illness began with classical Parkinson's disease the cognitive abnormality being a later development. Visual hallucinations of organic aetiology are notoriously difficult to treat as in this case.

Dementia with cerebral tumours

Aetiology

The prevalence of cerebral tumours increases with age, and in many series where the aetiology of the dementia syndrome has been carefully evaluated (for example Smith and Kiloh, 1981) are a relatively common cause of the dementia syndrome. The commonest are cerebral metastases (especially from lung), meningiomas and pituitary adenomas.

Clinical features

Where clear neurological symptoms and signs, such as raised intracranial pressure (headache, vomiting and papilloedema), epilepsy and cranial nerve palsies, exist the diagnosis of cerebral tumour is readily suggested. Yet many cerebral tumours are not recognized in old people and are found only at post-mortem (Walker et al., 1985).

Are these tumours really 'clinically silent'? The published evidence in fact suggests that the symptoms of cerebral tumour whilst not exactly 'loud' are there to be recognized in most cases. Those tumours which present with dementia as the main feature are usually gliomas or meningiomas, typically in frontal or mid-line areas, posterior fossa tumours are uncommon in old people. In such situations they are unlikely to be associated with symptoms of raised intracranial pressure, but are extremely likely to be associated with frontal lobe cognitive abnormalities or 'mild' cognitive impairment.

Malignant hemispheric tumours, either primary or metastatic, in old people usually present with progressive focal neurological deficit most often a hemiparesis but other include, dysphasia and visual field defects (Godfrey and Caird, 1984). Fluctuation of focal signs or episodic confusional states can occur and are often attributed to cerebrovascular disease. Cognitive impairment in these cases is usually of relatively short duration, 3 months to 2 years (Godfrey and Caird, 1984).

Meningiomas may be present for many years before diagnosis. They too may have fluctuation of symptoms and signs. In only a relatively small number of cases does dementia exists without 'focal' neurological signs, but many cases show signs of frontal lobe dysfunction (Riisoen and Fossan, 1986). Meningiomas in old people often present with recent decline in mental function irrespective of the length of the previous history.

The clinical features which suggest that cerebral tumour may be the underlying cause of the dementia syndrome are; relatively short history of cognitive impairment, progression of focal neurological signs, fluctuation in signs and symptoms, prominent frontal lobe signs.

Response to treatment

One of the problems for an old person with a cerebral tumour (apart from having the diagnosis made) is the apparent reluctance of some doctors to treat them. The published data do not support such a nihilistic approach. In malignant hemispheric tumours Godfrey and Caird (1984) found improvement in 50 per cent of patients treated with high dose steroids with a low incidence of side-effects and those cases reviewed by Byrne (1987) showed an overall improvement of 75 per cent in those treated. Although these benefits may be short lived, due presumably to the progression of malignancy, they enormously benefit the quality of life of the patient in their final months. In a proportion of patients with meningioma a complete recovery can occur following surgery.

> *A 65 year-old man had a gradual (over 6 months) change in his personality. He became disinihibited in his speech, swearing at neighbours and at times seemed quite depressed. He seemed to 'think slowly' according to his family. On assessment he had a sub-cortical dementia. There were no focal neurological signs apart from the evidence of frontal lobe signs (perseveration, difficulty in set-shifting, personality change and mood disorder). CT scan revealed a large frontal meningioma. He made an uneventful recovery from surgery.*

The history and examination in this case were consistent with a diagnosis of frontal lobe pathology. There is much debate as to what constitutes a 'focal' sign in the neurological examination. Some restrict the term to pyramidal signs whereas others (of whom I am one) include any clear evidence of lobar disfunction such as in this case.

Dementia with communicating hydrocephalus

Aetiology

The triad of symptoms dementia, ataxia and incontinence associated with impairment of resorption of cerebrospinal fluid in the arachnoid villi leading to hydrocephalus was first described by Hakim and Adams in 1965. They reported that the syndrome was associated with normal cerebrospinal fluid pressure, and hence came the name 'normal pressure hydrocephalus'. It is now known that some cases have rises in intracranial pressure especially at night. Its aetiology is unknown in the majority of cases but it may be secondary to conditions such as cerebral haemorrhage or head injury. Communicating hydrocephalus is the second commonest cause of reversible dementia (Byrne, 1987).

Clinical features

Cognitive changes are the initial feature and have a gradual onset. Typically they take the form of a sub-cortical dementia with prominent slowing of cognition and only mild forgetfulness associated with mood changes. In some cases these features are more pronounced in the mornings – what has been described as 'the fogged-in' feeling (Byrne, 1986). Ataxia is various in type, from gait apraxia to magnet gait (where the feet seem to stick to the floor after every step) to a vague unsteadiness, and emerges after the cognitive symptoms (occasionally they may occur at the same time). The urinary incontinence has been described as of the frontal type, where the patient is apparently unconcerned by the occurrence. Not all cases show the full triad of symptoms; some have predominant psychiatric symptoms (Price and Tucker, 1977).

Treatment

Is by diversion of Cerbrospinal fluid from the ventricles to the venous system or to the peritoneum by means of a shunt. There is disagreement as to the indications for surgery and those symptoms, which best predict outcome. Some advocate that patients with CT scan appearances suggestive of the condition–symmetrically enlarged ventricles with peri-ventricular lucency – should have intra-cranial pressure monitoring (Crockard et al., 1977). The finding of B waves on such recordings have a positive predictive association with treatment outcome. CSF outflow conductance studies-demonstrating failure of CSF circulation – are also associated with outcome, low conductance predicts a good outcome (Thomsen et al., 1986). Other features which have been associated with good response to treatment are; a known aetiology, the triad, and the presence of subcortical dementia (Thomsen., et al 1986; Black, 1980, Byrne, 1986).

A 76 year-old retired professor of physics was referred for reassessment after he had been diagnosed as having Alzheimer's disease. Until the age of 72 he was still working part-time and gave master classes in chess. He began to become mildly forgetful and complained he was 'slowing down'. He made mistakes in chess, largely because, as he put it, 'I seem to get stuck after a move or so'. He was assessed by a hospital specialist and told he had senile dementia. He asked if it was Alzheimer's disease and received an affirmative response. He began to use a stick as he became unsteady on his feet and in the last 6 months had become incontinent of urine. His wife did not think he had Alzheimer's disease and firmly requested reassessment.

When he was first seen he asked to 'be put down'. He was depressed but also showed sub-cortical dementia and gait apraxia. CT scan showed communicating hydrocephalus and a Dandy Walker syndrome. After a shunt operation he improved dramatically, became his former cheerful self, walked unaided, was continent and resumed his chess demonstrations.

At the time of the assessment this patient did not have the full triad of Hakim and Adams (1965). His cognitive impairment was even then, however, largely frontal and quite unlike Alzheimer's disease. One suspects that if he had been 66 rather than 74 when first seen he would have had a CT scan in the first place.

References

Alzheimer, A. (1907). Uber eine eigenartige erkrankung der hirnrinde. *Allgerneine zeitschrift fur psychiatria ind Psychisch-gerichtlick medicin*. **64**: 146–148.

Babikian, V. and Roppon, A.J. (1987). Binswanger's disease: a review. *Stroke*. **18**: 2.

Baddeley, A.D., Bressi, S., Della Sala, S., Logie, R. and Spinner, H. (1991). The decline of working memory in Alzheimer's disease. A longitudinal study. *Brain*. **114**, 2521–2542.

Black, P.M. (1980). Idiopathic normal pressure hydrocephalus: results of shunting 62 patients. *Journal of Neurosurgery* **52**: 371–377.

Blennow, K., Wallin, A. and Gottfries, C.G. (1991). Hetergeneity of 'probable Alzheimer's disease.' In *Alzheimer's Disease: Basic Mechanisms, Diagnosis and Therapeutic Strategies*. Igbal, K. et al. (eds). Chichester: Wiley, pp. 21–26.

Binswanger, O. (1984). Die abgrenzung der allgemeinen progressive paralyse. *Berliner Klinische Wochenshrift*. **32**: 1137–1139.

Burns, A., Jacoby, R. and Levy, R. (1990a). Psychiatric phenomena in Alzheimer's disease. 1: Disorders of thought content. *British Journal of Psychiatric*. **157**: 72–75.

Burns, A., Jacoby, R. and Levy, R. (1990b). Psychiatric phenomena in Alzheimer's disease. II: Disorders of thought content. *British Journal of Psychiatry*. **157**: 76–80.

Burns, A., Jacoby, R. and Levy, R. (1990c). Psychiatry Phenomena in Alzheimer's disease. III: Disorders of thought content. *British Journal of Psychiatry*. **157**: 81–85.

Burns, A., Jacoby, R. and Levy, R. (1990d). Psychiatric phenomena in Alzheimer's disease. IV: Disorders of thought content. *British Journal of Psychiatric* **157**: 86–94.

Byrne, E.J. (1986). The dementia study. In *Festschrift for Leslie Gadlon Kiloh*. University of New South Wales, pp. 123–138.

Byrne, E.J. (1987). Reversible dementia. *International Journal of Geriatric Psychiatry* **2**: 72–81.

Byrne, E.J. (1991). Diffuse Lewy body disease In *Recent advances in Psychogeriatrics*

Vol. 2. Arie, T. (ed.). Edinburgh: Churchill Livingstone, pp. 33–43.

Byrne, E.J. (1992). Diffuse Lewy Body disease: Disease, spectrum disorder or variety of Alzheimer's disease. *International Journal and Geriatric Psychiatry*. **7**: 229–324.

Byrne, E.J., Arie, T. (1991). Are drugs targeted at Alzheimer's disease useful? Insufficeint evidence of worthwhile benefit. In *Controversies in Therapeutics.Rubin, P. (ed.). London: British Medical Journal, pp. 50–51.*

Byrne, E.J., Lennox, G., Godwin-Austen, R.B. (1991a). Dementia associated with cortical Lewy bodies: proposed clinical diagnostic criteria. *Dementia*. **2**: 283–284.

Byrne, E.J., Lennox, G., Lowe, J. and Godwin-Austen, R.B. (1989). Diffuse Lewy body disease: clinical features in 15 cases. *Journal of Neurology, Neurosurgery and Psychiatry*. **52**: 709–717.

Byrne, E.J., Smith, C.W., Arie, T. (1991b). The diagnosis of dementia – I: Clinical and pathological criteria: A review of the literature. *International Journal of Geriatric Psychiatry* **6**: 199–208.

Chui, C., Teng, E.L., Henderson, V.W. and Moy, A.C. (1985). Clinical subtypes of dementia of the Alzheimer type. *Neurology* **35**: 1544–1550.

Chynoweth, R. and Foley, J. (1969). Pre-senile dementia responding to steroid therapy. *British Journal of Psychiatry*. **115**: 703–708.

Crockard, H.A., Hanlon, K., Duda, E.E. and Mullan, J.F. (1977). Hydrocephalus as a cause of dementia: evaluation by computerised tomography and intra cranial pressure monitoring. *Journal of Neurosurgery, Neurology and Psychiatry* **40**: 736–740.

Del Ser, T., Bermejo, F., Portera, A., Arredondo, J.M., Bouras, C., Constantinidis, J. (1990). Vascular dementia a clinicopathological study. *Journal of the Neurological Sciences*. **96**: 1–7.

Dennis, M.S., Byrne, E.J., Hopkinson, N. and Bendall, P (1992). Neurophyschiaric systemic lupus erythematosus in elderly people: a case series. *Journal of Neurology, Neurosurgery and Psychiatry*. **55**: 1157–1161.

Dickson, D.W., Wu, E., Crystal, H.A., Matthaiace, L.A., Yew, S-H.C., Davies, P. 1002. Alzheimer's disease and age related pathology in diffuse Lewy body disease. In: *Heterogeneity of Alzheimer's Disease*. Bolter, F. et al. (eds). Berlin/Heidelberg: Springer-Verlag pp. 169–186.

Eagger, S.A., Levy, R. and Saahakian. B.J. (1991). Tacrine in Alzheimer's disease. *Journal of the American Geriatrics Society* **33**: 167–169.

Ebrahim, S. (1990). *Clinical Epidemiology of Stroke*. Oxford: Oxford University Press.

Ettlin, T.E., Staehelin, H.B. and Kischka, U. (1989). Computed tomography, electroencephalography and clinical features in the differential diagnosis of senile dementia. *Archives of Neurology* **46**: 1217–1220.

Fenn, H., Luby, V., Yesavage, J.A. (1993). Subtypes in Alzheimer's disease and the impact of excess disability. Recent findings. *International Journal of Geriatric Psychiatry*. **8**: 67–74.

Fisher, C.M. (1965). Lacunes: small deep cerebral infarcts. *Neurology*. **15**: 774–784.

Fisher, C.M. (1982). Lacunar strokes and infarcts: A review. *Neurology*. **32**: 871–876.

Forstal, H., Burns, A., Luther, P., Cairns, N. and Levy, R. (1993). The Lewy body variant of Alzhimer's disease. Clinical and pathological findings. *British Journal of Psychiatry* **102**: 385–392.

Gibb, W.R.G., Esiri, M.M. and Lees, A.J. (1987). Clinical and pathological features of diffuse cortical Lewy body disease (Lewy body dementia). *Brain* **110**: 1131–1153.

Godfrey, J.B. and Caird, F.I. (1984). Intracranial tumous in the elderly: diagnosis and treatment. *Age and Ageing*. **13**: 152–158.

Gustafson, L. and Nilsson, L. (1982). Differential diagnosis of presenile dementia on clinical grounds. *Acta Psychiatrica Scandinavia*. **65**: 194.

Hachinski, V.C., Iliff, L.D., Zilka, E., Du Boulay, G.H., McAllister, V.L., Marshall, J. et al (1975). Cerebral blood flow in dementia. *Archives of Neurology*, **32**: 632–637.

Hachinski, V.C., Potter, P. and Merskey H. (1987). Leuko-ariosis. *Archives of Neurology*. **44**: 21–23.

Hakim, S. and Adams, R.D. (1965). The special clinical problems of symptomatic hydrocephalus with normal cerebral spinal fluid pressure. *Journal of Neurology, Neuro-surgery and psychiatry*. **2**: 302–327.

Hansen, L., Solman, D. and Galasko, D. (1990). The Lewy body variant of Alzheimer's disease: A clinical and patholgical entity. Neurology **40** 1–8.

Hart, S. and Semple, J. M. (1990). *Neuropsychology and the Dementias*. London: Taylor and Francis.

Henderson, V.W., Mack, W. and Williams, B.W. (1989). Spatial disorientation in Alzheimer's disease. *Archives of Neurology*. **46**: 391–394.

Heir, D.B., Warach, J.D., Gorelick, P.B., Thomas, J. (1989). Predictors of survival in clinically diagnosed Alzheimer's disease and multi-infarct dementia. *Archives of Neurology*. **46**: 1213–1216.

Hershey, L.A., Modic, M.T., Greenough, G. and Jaffe, D.G. (1987). Magnetic resonance imaging in vascular dementia. Neurology **37**: 29–36.

Janota, I, Mirsen, T.R., Hachinski, V.C., Lee, D.H., Henstay, H. (1989). Neuropathological correlates of leuko-araiosis. *Archives of Neurology*. **40**: 1124–1128.

Katona, C.L.E. (1989). Multi-infarct dementia In. *Dementia Disorders Advances and Prospects. Kantona, C. (ed.). London: Chapman and Hall, pp. 86–103*.

Katz, D.I., Alexander, M.P. and Mandell, A.M. (1987). Dementia following stroke in the mesencephalon and di-encephalon. *Archives of Neurology*. **44**: 1127–1133.

Katzman, R. (1985). Clinical presentation of the course of Alzheimer's disease: the atypical patient. *Interdisciplinary Topics in Gerontology*. **20**: 12–18.

Kirk, A. and Kertesz, A. (1991). On drawing impairment in Alzheimer's disease. *Archives of Neurology*. **48**: 73–77.

Kosaka, K. (1990). Diffuse Lewy body disease in Japan. *Journal of Neurology*. **237**: 197–204.

Levy, R. (1991). Are drugs targeted at Alzheimer's disease useful? Useful for what? In: Controversies in therapeutics (ed. P Rubin). British Medical Journal pp 49–50.

Lishman, W.A. (1987). *Organic Psychiatry*. 2nd edn. Oxford: Blackwell, pp 319–369.

Marie, P. (1901). Des joyers lacunaires de disinte.g.ration et de differents autres etats cavitaires du *Cerveau Nerue Medicine* (Paris) **32**: 281–298.

Medical Research Council Working Party (1992). MRC Trial of treatment of hypertension in older adults principal results. *British Medical Journal*. **304**; 405–412.

Meyer, J.S., Judd, B.W. and Tawaklna, T. (1986). Improved cognition after control of risk factors for multi-infarct dementia. *Journal of the American Geriatrics Society*. **256**: 2203–.

McKeith, I.G., Perry, R.H., Fairburn, A.F., Jabeen, S., Perry, E.K. (1993). Operational criteria for senile dementia of the Lewy body type (SDLT). *Psychological Medicine*.

Mielke, R., Hherholz, K., Grond, M., Kessler, J. and Heiss, W-D. (1992). Severity of vascular dementia is related to volume of metabolically impaired tissue. *Archives of Neurology.* **49**: 909–913.

Molsa, P.A., Marttila, R.J., Rinne, U.K. (1986). Survival and cause of death in Alzheimer's disease and multi-infarct dementia. *Acta Neurological Scandinavia.* **74**: 103–107.

Perry, R.H., Irving, D., Blessed, G., Fairbairn, A., Perry, E.K. (1990). Senile dementia of the Lewy body type. A clinically and neurolpathologically distinct form of Lewy body dementia. *Journal of the Neurological Sciences.* **95**: 119–139.

Price, T.R.P. and Tucker, G.J. (1977). Psychiatric and behavioural manifestations of normal pressure hydrocephalus. *Journal of Nervous and Mental Disease* **164**: 51–55.

Rapcsak, S.Z., Kentros, M. and Rubens. A.B. (1989). Impaired recognition of meaningful sounds in Alzheimer's disease. *Archives of Neurology.* **46**: 391–1300.

Riisoen, H and Fossan, G.O. (1985). How shall we investigate dementia to exclude intracronial meningiomas as a cause? An analysis of 34 patients with meningiomas. *Age and Ageing.* **15**: 29–34.

Roman, G.C., Tatemichi, T.K., Etunjuntti, T. et al. (1993). Vascular dementia: Diagnostic criteria for research studies. Report of the NINDS-AREN International workshop. *Neurology.* **43**: 250–260.

Rossor, M.N., Iversen, L.L., Reynolds, G.P., Mountjoy, C.Q. and Roth, M. (1984). Neurochemical characteristics of early and late onset types of Alzheimer's disease. *British Medical Journal.* **288**: 961–964.

Roth, M. and Wischik C.M. (1986). The heterogeneity of Alzheimer's disease and its implications for scientific investigations of the disorder. In. *Recent Advances in Psychogeriatrics. Arie, T. (ed.). Edinburgh: Churchill Livingstone, p. 71.*

Shuttleworth, E.C. (1984). Atypical presentations of dementia of the Alzheimer type. *Journal of the American Geriatric Society.* **32**: 485–490.

Smith, J.S. and Kiloh, L.G. (1981). This in vestigation of dementia: results in 200 consecutive admissions. *Lancet.* **1**: 824–827.

Steingart, A., Hachinski, V.C. and Lau, C. 1987. Cognitive and necrologic findings in subjects with diffuse white matter lucanes computed tomography scan (Leuko-araiosis) *Archives of Neurology.* **44**: 32–35.

Stienke, W., Sacco, R.L., Muhr, J.P., Foulkes, M.A., Tatemich, T.K., Wold, P.A, Price, T.R., Hitr, D.B. (1992). Thalamic stroke presentation and prognosis of infarcts and haemorrhages. *Achives of Neurology.* **49**: 703–710.

Thomsen, A.M., Borgesoin, S.E., Bruhn, P. and Gjerris, F. (1986). Prognosis of dementia in normal pressure hydrocephaslus after a shunt operation. *Annals of Neurology.* **20**: 304–310.

Tierney, M.C., Fisher, R.H., Lewis, A.J. (1988). The NINCDS – ADRDA work group. Alzheimer's disease. A clinico-pathological. *Neurology.* **38**: 359–364.

Tomlinson, B.E., Blessed, G. and Roth, M. (1968). Observations on the brains of non-demented old people. *Journal of Neurological Sciences.* **7**: 331–.

Tomlinson, B.E., Blessed, G. and Roth, M. (1970). Observations on the brains of demented old people. *Journal of Neurological Science.* **11**: 205–242.

Tupler, L.A., Coffey, E., Logue, P.E., Djang, W.T. and Fagan, S.M. (1992). Neuropsychological importance of subcortical white matter hyperintensity. *Archives of Neurology.* **49**: 1248–1252.

Ulrich, J., Probst, A. and Wuest, M. (1986). The brain diseases causing senile dementia. *Journal of Neurology.* **233**: 118–122.

Walker, A.E., Robins, M., Weinfield, F.A. (1985). Epidemiology of brain tumours. The national survey of intra-cranial neuroplasmas. *British Medical Journal.* **35**: 219–226.

Weisberg, L.A. (1982). Lacunar infarcts. Clinical and computed topographic correlations. *Archives of Neurology.* **39**: 37–40.

Welsh, K.A., Butters, N., Hughes, J.P., Mohs, R.C. and Heyman, A. (1992). Detection and staging in Alzheimer's disease. Use of the neuropsychological measures developed for the consortium to establish a register for Alzheimer's disease. *Archives of Neurology.* **49**: 448–452.

Williams, S.W., Byrne, E.J. and Stokes, P. (1993). Diffuse Lewy Body disease: An open trial of treatment in five cases. *International Journal of Geriatric Psychiatry* (in press).

Chapter 9 _____

The investigation of confusional states

Clinical investigations are used in two ways with respect to confusional states in old people: to ascertain the underlying cause, and to identify factors which may aggravate pre-existing cognitive impairment. Which clinical investigations should be used and whether all patients with confusional states should have a routine battery of tests are questions which have not been fully addressed. The following discussion will use what little data is available, but will mainly consist of pragmatic suggestions.

The investigation of delirium

Routine clinical investigations in delirium have been advocated by a number of authors, with a fair degree of agreement among them as to which tests should be included. What is lacking is information on the yield from such batteries. They do, however, have the merit of relating closely to the common aetiologies of delirium in old people. Table 9.1 shows the clinical investigations recommended as routine in the investigations of delirium in old people. The tests are grouped according to the level of agreement among the authors. Only one of the authors considers that a CT scan should be routine in the investigation of delirium, most consider it to be a second line investigation in selected cases.

Some consider that an EEG is the most useful investigation (Liston, 1982;

Table 9.1 Recommended routine investigations in delirium

All
   FBC, ESR
   Blood chemistry – electrolytes, calcium, phosphate, LFTs, glucose

All but one
   Serology for syphilis
   EEG
   TFT
   Urea, creatinine

Sources: Beresin (1988), Lindesay et al. (1990), Lipowski (1992).

Lipowski, 1992), as abnormalities, such as diffuse slowing, are inevitably present and correlate with the degree of arousal and cognitive impairment of the patient. Others point out that diffuse slowing is also a feature of many diseases that cause dementia (Lindesay et al., 1990) and because the two syndromes frequently co-exist, this lessens its usefulness.

There is also an important practical problem – that of requiring the patient to lie still for about 20 minutes (Leuchter and Jacobson, 1991). There is some evidence that more powerful EEG techniques, such as quantitative EEG (where the electrical activity is recorded digitally and spectral power analysed by computer) are more discriminating and have the great advantage of being much faster than conventional EEG.

The inclusion by some authors of serology for syphilis as a routine investigative test for delirium must be questioned. While neurosyphilis still exists it is rare.

All agree that other tests (see Table 9.2), should be selective according to the history, examination and results of the routine battery. A surprising omission from these select investigations are simple tests of pulmonary function, such as peak flow, as chronic obstructive airways disease (COAD) is commonly associated with cognitive dysfunction and respiratory disorders are a common aggravating factor in dementia (often leading to delirium). With the exception of the chest X-ray (and possibly the ECG) this routine battery can be performed wherever the patient is located.

Using similar batteries of tests, two recent prospective studies of delirium in hospitalized old people were able to identify the probable causes in most cases (Francis et al. 1990; Koponen Riekkinen, 1993). In one of these studies, however, (Francis et al., 1990) multiple aetiology was very common occurring in 22 out of 50 patients (44 per cent).

Such a routine battery is also relatively inexpensive (currently about £80). The cost-benefit ratio cannot be calculated as adequate information on yield is not available, it is likely to be favourable given the low cost of the battery

Table 9.2 Selective investigations for delirium

Screen for drugs and alcohol
Arterial blood gases
Serum-Mg, B12 and folate, proteins, osmolality
Blood culture
Anti-nuclear antibody
CSF analysis
White cell scan
Echocardiogram
Ultrasound
TFT
CT

Sources: Beresin (1988), Lindesay et al. (1990), Lipowski (1992)

the common occurrence of the syndrome and the high morbidity in untreated cases.

The investigation of dementia

The use of investigations in dementia has been extensively reviewed (e.g. Siu, 1991;, Byrne et al., 1992). Despite this there is still little information on which tests to use and whether or not they should be routine. Routine investigation of the dementia syndrome is advocated by some for all patients as they argue that it is important not to miss any reversible causes. While I agree with that sentiment, it is apparent that we are still taking a rather blunderbuss approach to investigations and that important questions which might help to focus our approach are often not considered. First, how many of the tests that are commonly recommended in routine test batteries actually are diagnostic of the underlying cause of the dementia syndrome? The answer is very few (Byrne et al., 1992) and there is little data on the yield of such tests (Larson et al., 1986). Second, what are we looking for when we say that we are seeking reversible causes? The answer seems to be that we are looking for different things; for example, some include alcohol as a reversible dementia whereas others do not. Finally, although dementia syndrome is commoner in old age, few have reported the frequency of reversible causes according to age.

What is needed is a reconsideration of the use of such routine test batteries in order to address the issues raised above. Until such data is available I, like many others, probably over-investigate. There are some guidelines available which could usefully be considered.

The Canadians have taken a novel approach to these issues by making a careful examination of the prevalence of the diseases which may cause dementia, their degree of reversibility and the importance of diagnosing them, and assign a degree of priority to each (Canadian Consensus Conference, 1989). With colleagues, I surveyed hospital specialists (geriatric medicine, psychiatry, neurology and psychiatry of old age) to ascertain their current practise in the use of routine investigations (Byrne et al., 1992). The specialists in this study were being selective in their use of routine investigation especially in the very old. Their use of routine tests in patients aged 65–74 years and in those aged 75–84 years or more is shown in Figs 9.1 and 9.2. Overall the old-age specialists use more investigations routinely, but their routine use of these investigations was influenced by the age of the patient – the oldest patients (85+ years) had the fewest tests. In this study we considered the test battery recommended by authorities in the field, shown in Table 9.3, and compared it to the hospital specialists battery. Although there was close agreement between them for those aged <65 years and 65–74 years, the

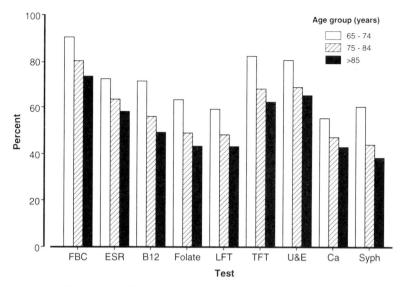

Source: Unpublished data Byrne et al. (1992).

Fig. 9.1   Use of blood tests by hospital specialists as part of routine screen or the investigation of dementia syndrome

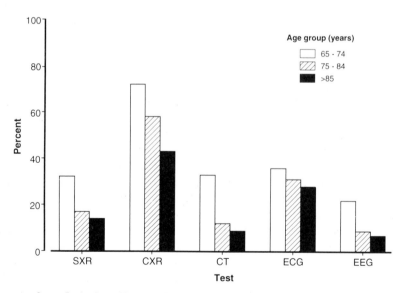

Source: Previously unpublished data Byrne et al. (1992).

Fig. 9.2   Use of radiological and other investigations by hospital specialists as part of the investigation of the dementia syndrome

Table 9.3 'Recommended' tests in the investigation of the dementia syndrome

---

Full blood count
B_{12}
Folate
Thyroid function
Urea and electrolytes
Calcium
Liver function tests
Computed topographic scan
Erythrocyte sedimentation rate
Serology for syphilis

Source: Byrne et al. (1992)

hospital specialists were much more selective in investigating routinely the 'old' old.

Such 'recommended' test batteries are not of universal application. For example, in Sweden there is a relatively high incidence of Borrelia which can affect the CNS and is tested for routinely by some Swedish centres (Wallin and Blennow, 1992). Although all the tests can be performed in most health district's hospitals, some laboratories will not perform some tests routinely, for example serum B12 unless there are haematological changes. (That the CNS can be affected by B12 deficiency in the absence of haematological change has been established in a few cases (Gross et al., 1986).)

Perhaps the most contentious test is the CT scan. There are those who advocate its routine use in all patients (NIA, 1980) and those who argue for a more selective use (Arie, 1985). It is the single most expensive test in the 'recommended' battery. There are a number of published clinical prediction rules (see review by Martin et al., 1987) which can assist in the selection of patients to scan, but all have relatively high misclassification rates – that is, too many potentially treatable lesions are missed. Until this issue is resolved one pragmatic approach is to scan all patients under 65 years (and probably under 70 years) who present with relatively acute onset, or with 'atypical ' features. This approach has yet to be critically assessed.

It is likely that the greatest yield from these tests is information about aggravating factors rather than information directly relating to the aetiology of the syndrome. This is of no small import as adjustments in homeostasis in the elderly patient with dementia can lead to beneficial, measurable and functionally relevant improvement. The extent to which this occurs is not yet established, although there is a little information. Larson et al. 1986 found that few of the abnormal results in either selective testing or in routine testing of patients with dementia were clinically relevant, but that a few tests were useful in detecting aggravating factors (or unsuspected disease); full blood count, thyroid function tests, and blood chemistry, especially sodium, calcium and glucose. Colgan and Philpott 1985 examined the routine use of investigations in psychogeriatric patients and also found that FBC and blood chemistry detected abnormalities that could be acted upon, as did serum folate and urinalysis. What is lacking in these studies is information on the outcome of treating the patients having established an abnormality or abnormalities. My clinical impression is that it is of benefit, but that is a hypothesis to be tested!

There is some evidence that some of the newer imaging techniques such as nuclear magnetic resonance may assist in distinguishing between the common aetiological causes of dementia – Alzheimer's disease, vascular dementia, but they are at present a relatively scarce resource.

Determining the aetiology of the dementia syndrome in a particular case is important and is likely to be more so for two main reasons; carers (and some sufferers) want to know, and effective treatments for degenerative diseases are now theoretically possible.

Until the definitive tests appear it is probably cost effective to over- rather than to under-investigate. The cost of the 'recommended' test battery is about £40–£50 (excluding CT scant). To investigate all new cases of the dementia syndrome in a health district each year, around 700 (based on incidence data from Nottingham–Morgan et al., 1992) would cost £28,000–£35,000. One would only need to identify one or two cases of reversible dementia (and one would expect somewhat more) with the savings to the health and social services this represents to produce a favourable cost:benefit ratio.

The investigation of other confusional states

There are no widely recommended batteries of investigations for the assessment of other confusional states in old people. Important considerations are: knowledge of the common physical illnesses (and some uncommon ones) that may present with psychiatric syndromes; psychiatric illness may be a reaction (or a temporally related) to physical illness of any kind; physical illness may exist coincidentally with psychiatric illness and the side-effects of drugs may include psychiatric disorders.

Depression

In the absence of a previous history of depression, or of a family history of depression, depression with onset in old age is frequently the symptom of an underlying occult physical disorder. Some of the diseases which may present with depression as the first or major symptom in old age are shown in Table 9.4.

Both intracerebral and extracerebral tumours may present with depression, the mechanism in the latter being unknown. Thyroid disease in old people may present with few of the typical features, whether hypo- or hyperfunction

Table 9.4 Conditions which may present with depression in old people

---

Tumour: intracerebral, extracerebral
Metabolic: hypercalcaemia (primary or secondary), renal or hepatic failure
Endochrine: hypo or hyperthyroidism
Infection: non-specific effect of any infection-specific, neurosyphilis
Cardiovascular: occur myocardial infection
Connective tissue disorders: systemic lupus erythematosus (SLE)
Degenerative: Parkinson's disease
Cerebrovascular: stroke
Miscellaneous: communicating hydrocephalus, pernicious anaemia, alcohol dependence

---

is involved. Neurosyphilis is rare but may present with depression or dementia. Disorders of circulation may occasionally present with depression and depressive illnesses have a high mortality from cardiovascular disease (Murphy et al., 1988). Up to 40 per cent of patients with Parkinson's disease have depression before the onset of obvious motor symptoms but is perhaps more common as a sequelae than as a presentation. Systemic lupus erythematosus (SLE) was thought to be rare in old people but some recent series suggest that it is in fact not uncommon and can present with depression (Dennis et al., 1992). Occasionally depression or apathy can be a presentation of hypothermia in old people.

From these observations a routine battery of tests can be suggested, as shown in Table 9.5. This is an empirical approach which requires validation.

Table 9.5 Suggested routine investigations for depression of late onset

---

Blood tests: FBC, ESR, U&E, calcium, LFT, TFT
Others: ECGs, CXR

Other psychiatric disorders

Paranoid states on late onset

In about one-third of such cases there is associated organic disease (Post, 1966; Holden, 1987), often intracerebral of which the commonest are cerebrovascular disease and degenerative neurological disorders (Huntington's chorea, Alzheimer's disease, diffuse Lewy body disease). Such degenerative changes are perforce mild or at an early stage, as a degree of cortical sparing is required to produce paranoid symptoms (Cummings, 1985). Even in cases with no symptoms of intracerebral disease, cognitive abnormalities and enlargement of the cerebral ventricles have been demonstrated when compared to normal elderly people (Naguib and Levy,

1987). Deafness or other sensory impairment may exacerbate the symptoms in such cases (Naguib and Levy, 1987).

Anxiety

Pure anxiety states in old people occur in about 3 per cent of the population aged 65 years or more. Anxiety is more commonly seen in association with depression and its investigation should perhaps be similar to the scheme suggested above. In a number of conditions anxiety may be the presenting feature, such as cardiovascular disease (infarction, arrhythmias) or endocrine disease (Hyperthyroidism). Anxiety is a common psychological reaction to existing physical disease of any kind. The severity of that illness is perhaps not as import as the patient's perception of threat – to their full independence in particular. Anxiety and depression may be presenting features of alcohol abuse in old people and conversely alcohol abuse may arise in old age as a consequence of these disorders in the setting of social isolation (Hodgson and Jolley 1986).

References

Arie, T. (1985). Dementia in the elderly In *Medicine in Old Age 2nd edn. London: British Medical Association, pp. 1–10.*

Beresin, E.V. (1988). Delirium in the elderly. *Journal of Geriatric Psychiatry and Neurology.* **1**: 127–143.

Byrne, E.J., Smith, C.W. Arie, T. and Lilley, J. (1992). Diagnosis of dementia 3 – Use of investigations. A survey of current consultant practice review of the literature and implications for audit. *International Journal of Geriatric Psychiatry.* **7**: 647–657.

Canadian Consensus Conference. (1989) The assessment of Dementia. Montreal.

Colgan, J. and Philpott, M. (1985). The routine use of investigations in elderly psychiatric patients. *Age and Ageing.* **14**: 163–167.

Cummings, J. (1985). Organic delusions: phenomenology, anatomical correlations and reviews. *British Journal of Psychiatry* **146**: 184–197.

Dennis, M.A., Byrne, E.J., Hopkinson, N. and Bendall, P. (1992). Neuropsychiatric systemic lupus erythematosus in elderly people: a case series. *Journal of Neurology, Neurosurgery and Psychiatry.* **55**: 1157–1161.

Francis, J., Martin, D. and Kapoor, W.N. (1990). A prospective study of delirium in hospitalised elderly. *Journal of the American Medical Association.* **263**: 1097–1101.

Gross, J.S., Weintraub, N.T., Neufeld, R.R. and Libow, L.S. (1986). Pernicious anaemics in the demented patient without anaemia or macrocytosis. A case for early recognition. *Journal of the American Geriatric Society.* **34**: 612–614.

Holden, N. (1987). Late paraphrenia or the paraphrenias? *British Journal of Psychiatry* **150**: 635–639.

Koponen, H.J. and Riekkinen, P.J. (1993). A prospective study of delirium in elderly patients admitted to a psychiatric hospital. *Psychological Medicine.* **23**: 103–109.

Larson, E.B., Reifler, B.V., Sumi, S.M., Confield, C.G. and Chinn, N.M. (1986). Diagnostic tests in the evaluation of dementia. A prospective study of 200 elderly out patients. *Archives of Internal Medicine*. **146**: 1917–1922.

Leuchter, A.F., Jacobson, S.A. (1991). Quantitative measurement of brain electrical activity in delirium. *International Psychogeriatrics* **3**: 231–247.

Lindsay, J. MacDonald, A. and Starke, I. (1990). The management of delirium In *Delirium in the elderly*. Oxford: Oxford University Press, pp. 88–89.

Lipowski, Z.J. (1992). Delirium and impaired consciousness. In *Oxford Textbook of Geriatric medicine. Evans, J.G. and Williams, T.F. (eds). Oxford: Oxford University Press. pp. 490–596.*

Liston, E.H. (1982). Delirium in the aged. *Psychiatric clinics of North America*. **5**: 49–66.

Martin, D.C., Miller, J., Kapoor, W., Karpf, M. and Boller, F. (1987). Clinical predication rules for computed topographic scanning in senile dementia. *Archives of Internal Medicine* **147**: 77–80.

Murphy, E., Smith, R., Lindesay, J. and Slattery, J (1988). Increased mortality rates in late-life depression. *British Journal of Psychiatry* **152**: 347–353.

Morgan, K., Lilley, J., Arie, T., Byrne, J. Jones, R and Waite, J. (1992). Incidence of dementia: preliminary findings from the Nottingham Longitudinal study of activity and ageing. *Neuroepidemiology* **11** (Suppl. 1) 80–83.

National Institute In Ageing Task Force (1980). Senility reconsidered: treatment possibilities for mental impairment in the elderly. *Journal of the American Medical Association* **24**: 259–263.

Naquib, M. and Levy, R. (1987). Late paraphrenia – neuro psychological impairment and structural brain abnormalities on computed tomography. *International Journal of Geriatric Psychiatry* **2**: 83–90.

Post, F. (1966). *Persistent Persecutory States of the Elderly*. Oxford: Pergamon.

Sui, A.L. (1991). Screening for dementia and investigating its causes. *Annals of Internal Medicine* **115**: 122–132.

Wallin, A. and Blennow, K. (1992). Clinical diagnosis of Alzheimer's disease by primary care physicians and specialists. *Acta Neurologica Scandinavica*, Suppl. **139**: 26–32.

Chapter 10 _____

Management of confusional states in old people

This chapter, rather than being all inclusive, will take a problem orientated approach. Useful and comprehensive discussions of the management of the major confusional states in old people can be found in the following: for dementia Arie (1986), Byrne and Arie (1990), for delirium Lipowski (1990), Macdonald et al. (1989), for depression Baldwin (1991).

General principles of management include; identifying the underlying cause and treatment of the cause or of the symptoms. identification of the needs (practical, physical, social) of both sufferer and carer, the use of drugs, the environment for management. Figures 10.1–10.3 show in schematic form the general management considerations for the three common confusional states in old people.

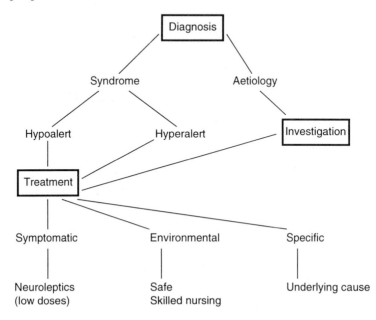

Fig. 10.1 Management of delirium

The management of behavioural change in confusional states

The successful management of behavioural change in confusional states in old people requires an understanding of the nature of the behaviour and its effect on others. Such an understanding can be reached by consideration of the following points.

1. *Behaviour can be disturbed or disturbing* Some behaviours in themselves are inherently likely to cause problems and can thus be described as disturbed. Severe physical aggression, persistent shouting or screaming are two examples. The nature of these behaviours is such that they are unlikely to be tolerated for long even in the most sympathetic surroundings and by the most sympathetic observers. The first is dangerous the second is extremely wearing.

   Other behaviours are not in themselves particularly disturbed, but may be perceived as such in certain settings. In certain environments, however, these same behaviours may be tolerated and considered safe.

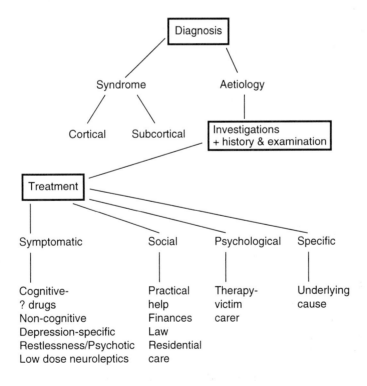

Fig. 10.2 Management of dementia

Thus whether the behaviour is disturbing depends on the observer and on the environment.

2. *Behaviour related to the disease process?*   It is sometimes assumed that all behavioural disturbance arising in confusional states are a result of the underlying disease process and are therefore less amenable to intervention. While behavioural changes are a common sequelae of disease, they may also be due to extrinsic factors or discomfort-symptoms of disease or of dis-ease. Before assuming that a behaviour is a symptom of the former, a careful assessment of factors that may lead to dis-ease should be made. Some of these factors are shown in Table 10.1, which is not an all inclusive list but is intended as a guide to such an assessment. Old people with cognitive impairment may be unable to communicate distress other than by a change in behaviour. Although some of the factors in Table 10.1., such as constipation, are well known others – such as the psychological reaction to being cognitively impaired – are perhaps less well appreciated and are denied by some. It has been assumed that people with Alzheimer's disease have 'no insight' and are therefore untroubled by their failing cognition. Some (Reisburg et al. 1982) takes issue with this long-held assumption and suggests that some patients are

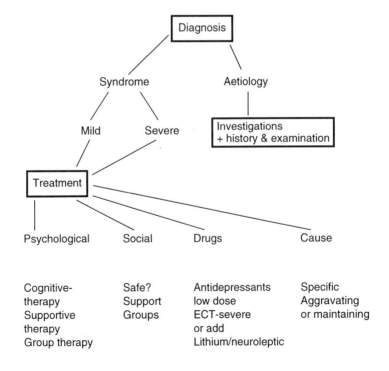

Fig. 10.3   Management of depression

Table 10.1 Some factors which may cause change in behaviour in patients with dementia (various aetiologies).

Physical illness	In any system. Common examples: infection, stroke, heart failure Delirium may be superimposed in dementia
Discomfort	Pain, wetness, constipation
Environment	Excessive noise, extremes of temperature, changes in the environment (e.g. a move)
Sensory impairment	Sight, hearing
Treatment	Drugs, especially antidepressants, anti-Parkinsonian agents
Alcohol	Even small amounts
Psychological factors	Anxiety, depression, psychotic experiences, anger, frustration, insight into failing cognition

Source: Byrne and Arie (1990). Reproduced with permission.

extremely troubled, albeit often in a fragmentary or transient fashion, by their failings.

3. *What is the behaviour?*   Close observation of 'wanderers' reveals that this term covers a wide variety of behaviour (Hope and Fairburn 1990). In some patients it appears to be aimless or part of a general over-arousal, in others it may appear purposeful although the purpose may be inappropriate, such as in the second of the examples below where the patient wants to go home to the home of his childhood. It is always important to assess a behaviour in detail using a scheme, for example: what is the patient actually doing; when are they doing it; where are they doing it; and to whom are they doing it? Appropriate intervention depends on the above considerations and is summarized in Table 10.2. Despite such a careful approach there are some problems that have no solutions, but it is always worth trying.

Table 10.2 Summary of management scheme for behavioural change in old people with confusional states

Observe the behaviour	What is it?
	When is it happening?
	Where is it happening?
	To whom is it happening?
Observe the patient	Disease or dis-ease?
Observe the environment	Safe?
	Contributing to the behaviour
Observe the observer	Is the behaviour a problem in the eye of the beholder?

An 86 year-old widow, known to her GP as having dementia, who lived alone and who had no relatives was repeatedly wandering around her neighbourhood. She never went far, but often knocked on her neighbours doors (at all hours of the day and night) to ask the time or for tasks to be done. Home assessment revealed dementia of the Alzheimer type. There were signs of considerable self-neglect in herself and her home was less than clean. Her neighbours were vociferous in their demands that something should be done!

The behaviour in this case could not be closely observed, but from the reports was in itself not very disturbed, rather it was disturbing the observers – in this case, the neighbours. There was no particular time for the behaviour's occurrence and her immediate environment was reasonably safe (she lived in a very quiet residential area). She was pale and dishevelled and showed signs of recent weight loss and in some dis-ease.

She refused to come to hospital either as a day or an in-patient, but did accept visits from domiciliary services and the community psychiatric nurse. On each visit the nurse saw the neighbours, to explain and to listen to their concerns. After about two months' she agreed to come to the day hospital. Here she was found to be anaemic-iron deficiency. She did not wander in the day hospital and with correction her anaemia and increased social support the wandering diminished very considerably. She remained at home for 2 years until she fell and fractured her left femur and was admitted to hospital. She died shortly afterwards.

A 76 year-old man was admitted to a geriatric medical ward with a chest infection. He had vascular dementia and was cared for at home, with no help from statutory services, by his wife. On the ward he was continually getting out of bed and making for the door saying he was going home. Home, however, was his childhood home, he said he had to get his father's tea. On two occasions he managed to leave the ward and became quite angry at being brought back.

The behaviour in this case was 'purposeful' but based on a different reality to that of the observers. It was noted to be most marked at night and, because there were fewer staff on the ward at that time, to be very troublesome and wearing. Close observation of the patient showed that at the time of the worst wandering he was more breathless. Peak flow readings before and after salbutomol inhalation showed reversible airways disease. He was commenced on regular nebulized salbutomol and a small dose of neuroleptic at night.

Although he still wandered for a few days he was quite amenable to persuasion. As his respiratory function improved so the behaviour ceased. He was discharged home to the care of his wife, with supervision from the hospital team. More support was needed as he grew more frail, but he died peacefully in his sleep at home one year later.

An outbreak of wandering among the patients with dementia on a psychogeriatric ward was solved by ice cold lemonade in large doses and the installation of 6 fans. The temperature on the ward was 100 degrees Fahrenheit!

The use of medication in management of confusional states in old people

Even when the most careful assessments are made of behaviour in old people with confusional states, not all behaviours respond to environmental measures, psychological support or the treatment of aggravating causes. In addition, some of the symptoms of confusional states, such as delusions or hallucinations, may be so troublesome as to warrant intervention.

Behaviour which arises in the setting of a generalized state of hyper-arousal, such as restlessness, agitation, aggression or sexual dis-inhibition may be amenable to neuroleptic medication. The obvious questions about the use of medication in such cases is which drug and what dose? There has been little careful evaluation comparing the efficacy of different neuroleptics for clearly defined problems of this type, and so their use is largely empirical. Some, such as chlorpromazine, are sedating but also have a high incidence of adverse effects, others, such as thioridazine, are less likely to produce extra-pyramidal side-effects but more likely to induce anti-cholinergic effects.

Most neuroleptics can be effective in doses which some consider 'homeopathic', and in such quantities are less likely to induce adverse effects. The newer neuroleptics, such as clozapine, are even more effective and are less likely to induce extrapyramidal symptoms, but they are expensive and have a high rate of blood dyscrasia. Neuroleptics have been shown to be useful in the treatment of hyper-arousal states with associated behavioural change (Liebovici and Tariot, 1988). Suggested dose levels are shown in Table 10.3.

Other drugs which may be useful for the treatment of hyper-arousal states are promazine 25–100 mg per day, fentazine 2–8 mg per day and chlormethiazole 500 mg-2 gms at night.

The treatment with drugs of symptoms of confusional states can also be seen as empirical. One such approach is to consider the symptom profile in

Table 10.3 Suggested dosage of different neuroeptics in the treatment of behaviour or of symptoms in confusional states in old people

Neuroleptic	Dose (start/maximum)
Thioridazine	10 mg, 2–3 times per day
	50 mg/day
Haloperidol	0.25 mg–0.5 mg, 1–2 per day
	3–5 mg per day
Chlorpromazine	25 mg, 1–3 times per day
	150 mg per day
Trifluoperazine	1 mg, 1–2 per day
	5 mg per day

those with cognitive disorders and use appropriate medication. For example, the old person with dementia who is apathetic and socially withdrawn, is behaviourally depressed and may be treated as if they had a functional depressive illness (Byrne and Arie, 1990; Leibovici and Tariot, 1988)

Treatment of symptoms in confusional states

An 86 year-old woman with dementia of the Alzheimer type was a resident in a nursing home. She spent most of the day in an agitated state, sometimes wandering around the home picking up objects, sometimes standing still looking preoccupied and wringing her hands. She had a permanent worried frown. Her dysphasic speech occasionally betrayed 'depressed' cognition ('It's awful', 'It's bad'). A 10 mg dose of amitriptyline at night created a woman more at peace with herself. She looked unperturbed, the frown disappeared and she was less restless.

An 88 year-old man developed a delirium in association with a urinary tract infection, previous cognitive impairment and deafness. He believed that the nurses were trying to poison him and he seemed to be hearing voices and seeing men in his room. The batteries in his hearing aid were replaced and he accepted medication in syrup form (thioridazine 10 mg b.d.) from his wife and subsequently from the nursing staff, with benefit.

The administration of medication to patients with confusional states is often a problem and raises some ethical and legal issues. Ethically any patient has the right to refuse medication or physical treatment. Legally doctors may only 'force' patients to take medication against their will if that patient fulfils the requirements of the Mental Health Act 1983 – that is they should be mentally ill and a danger to themselves or others and no other arrangements for their safe care can reasonably be made. Such medication may also only be to treat the mental state. The Mental Health Act does not allow treatment of physical illness. Although the patient mentioned above fulfiled the requirements of The Mental Health Act, the Act did not, and indeed only very rarely in such situations does it ever, need to be invoked. The staff on the ward asked the patient's wife to help. In other cases a flexible approach to the timing of medication administration pays dividends, for example, give the medication when the patient is settled, rather than sticking to the 12 o'clock dose. Some relatives give medication in the patient's tea or food. Although for health care staff this is unethical according to the principle of autonomy, it may be ethical according to the principle of beneficence, where the patients autonomy is compromised by cognitive impairment. There are no easy prescriptions for this ethical dilemma but the reader may be helped by reference to extensive discussions by Beauchamp and Childress (1989) and Oppenheimer (1991). As a general principle respect the patients wishes and try again.

References

Arie, T. (1986). Management of dementia: a review. *British Medical Bulletin.* **42**: 91–96.
Baldwin, R. (1991). Depressive illness. In *Psychiatry in the Elderly. Jacoby, R. and*

Oppenheimer, C. (eds). *Oxford: Oxford University Press pp. 676–719.*

Beauchamp, T.L. and Childress, J.F. (1989). *Principles of biomedical Ethics, 3rd edn. Oxford: Oxford University Press.*

Byrne, E.J. and Arie, T. (1990). Coping with dementia in the elderly. In *Current Medicine I*. Lawson, D.H. (ed.). Edinburgh: Churchill Livingstone, pp. 137–155.

Byrne, E.J., Arie, T. (1990). Coping with dementia. In *Current Medicine 2*. Lawson, D. (ed.). Edinburgh: Churchill Livingstone, pp. 137–155.

Hope, R.A., Fairburn, C.G. (1990). The nature of wandering in dementia in a community based study. *International Journal of Geriatric Psychiatry.* **5**: 239–245.

Leibovici, A. and Tariot, P.N. (1988). Agitation associated with dementia: systematic approach to treatment. *Psychopharmacology Bulletin* **24**: 49–53.

Lipowski, Z.J. (1990). *Delirium: Acute Confusional States.* New York: Oxford University Press.

MacDonald, A.J.D., Simpson, A. and Jenkins, D. (1989). Delirium in the elderly: review and a suggestion for a research programme. *International Journal of Geriatric Psychiatry.* **4**: 311–319.

Oppenheimer, C. (1991). Ethics and the psychiatry of old age. In *Psychiatry in the Elderly. Jacoby, R. and Oppenheimer, C. (eds). Oxford: Oxford University Press, pp. 940–950.*

Reisbury, B., Ferris, S.H., De Lean, M.J. and Crook, T. (1982). The global deterioration scale for assessment of primary degenerative dementia. *American Journal of Psychiatry* **139**: 1136–1139.

Reisberg, B., Ferris, S.H., De Lean, M.J. and Crook, T. (1982). The global deterioration scale for assessment of primary degenerative dementia. *American Journal of Psychiatry* **139**: 1136–1139.

Index